Population Politics and Development

Population Politics and Development

From the Policies to the Clinics

Lisa Ann Richey

palgrave
macmillan

POPULATION POLITICS AND DEVELOPMENT

First published in 2008 by
PALGRAVE MACMILLAN™
175 Fifth Avenue, New York, N.Y. 10010 and
Houndmills, Basingstoke, Hampshire, England RG21 6XS
Companies and representatives throughout the world.

PALGRAVE MACMILLAN is the global academic imprint of the Palgrave Macmillan division of St. Martin's Press, LLC and of Palgrave Macmillan Ltd. Macmillan® is a registered trademark in the United States, United Kingdom and other countries. Palgrave is a registered trademark in the European Union and other countries.

ISBN-13: 978–0–230–60292–2
ISBN-10: 0–230–60292–4

Library of Congress Cataloging-in-Publication Data

Richey, Lisa Ann.
Population politics and development : from the policies to the clinics / Lisa Ann Richey.
p. cm.
Includes bibliographical references and index.
ISBN 0–230–60292–4
1. Birth control—Tanzania. 2. Tanzania—Population policy. 3. Women in development—Tanzania. 4. Birth control—Africa. I. Title.

HQ766.5.T34R53 2008
304.6′6609678—dc22 2007025114

A catalogue record for this book is available from the British Library.

Design by Newgen Imaging Systems (P) Ltd., Chennai, India.

First edition: February 2008

10 9 8 7 6 5 4 3 2 1

Printed in the United States of America.

To my father William Hobson Richey (1930–2007)

Contents

List of Figures, Photos, and Tables

Figures

Photos

Tables

Acknowledgments

I have received many forms of support from individuals and institutions during the research and writing of this book and it is a pleasure to acknowledge them here. First, I would like to thank Ms. Perpetua Dyumyeko, Ms. Sarah Kwayu, Mr. Charles A.A. Moshi, Ms. Lily Makalanga, Ms. Hellen Masatu, Mr. Willy Mduma, Ms. Frida Mfinanga, Mr. Fredrick Mghase, Mr. Godgrace Moshi, Ms. Patricia Mugusie, Mr. Tumsifu Mushi, Ms. Asteria Mwatagu, Ms. Ida Ngoda, Mr. Rogness Swai for research assistance in Tanzania. I thankfully acknowledge financial support for various parts of this project from the J. William Fulbright Foundation, the Royster Society of Fellows, the Andrew W. Mellon Foundation, and the Danish Social Science Research Council. I am grateful to UTAFITI (the National Scientific Research Council of Tanzania) for granting and renewing research clearances, and to the regional, district, and village level government officials who permitted me to conduct fieldwork in areas under their jurisdiction. I wish to thank Dr. F.M. Mburu, Dr. Anne Fleuret, and Josselyn Neukom of the United States Agency for International Development (USAID/Tanzania); Mr. Bill Musoke, Mrs. Dorothy Temu-Usiri, and Mr. Chris Mwaijonga of UNFPA; Dr. E.P.Y. Muhondwa, of The Population Council; and Dr. Naomi Katunzi and Dr. Tengio Urrio of UMATI for granting me permission to conduct research in UMATI clinics and projects. I also acknowledge the International Planned Parenthood Federation (IPPF) London for access to their archives in the earliest stages of this work.

Many thanks are owed to Tanzanian public servants at all levels including: Mr. S.B. Buberwa, Mr. U.P.K. Tenende, the members of the Population Planning Unit in the Planning Commission; Dr. Calista Simbakalia, Dr. Catherine Sanga, Mr. Peter Riwa, and the staff of the Family Planning/Reproductive and Child Health Unit in the Ministry of Health; Mr. Sylvester Ngallaba, Mrs. A. Komba, and the staff at the Bureau of Statistics. At the University of Dar es Salaam, I thank Professor Rwekaza S. Mukandala, Professor Joe Lugalla, Professor C. Lwechungura Kamuzora, Sister Anita, and the members of the Women's Research and Documentation Project, and Professor Yunus Rubanza. Most of all, I am grateful for the friendship, intellectual, and logistical support from Professors Daudi and Fenella Mukangara.

In the regions where I worked, I am particularly thankful to all of the clinic officers, family planning service providers, and CBDs who patiently tolerated my presence in the midst of their work, and who taught me far more than I have been able to adequately express about the tribulations of health care provision in Tanzania. I am also most indebted to the many women who patiently shared important and intimate aspects of their experiences with me. In Morogoro Region, I would like to thank the Development Studies Institute at Sokoine University of Agriculture. I am grateful to the regional, district, and village medical staff including Amadeus Mwananziche, Dr. F. Fupi, Mrs. Margaret Wapalila, Mrs. S. Sabaya, Mrs. Maro and Mrs. Rupia and Mr. Alphonse Mkini and Mr. Greyson Chagama of UMATI. In Ruvuma, I thank Father Bonaventura Ndimbo and the late Father Vincent Tiwinga, the members of the Songea Development Action Project (SODA) and the regional, district, and village medical staff Dr. S.R. Kabuma, Mrs. Mwingira, Mrs. Mwidasi, Mrs. Rose Nylenda, and Mrs. Eli Munda Komba, and especially Dr. John Budotela for continuing support. In Kilimanjaro Region, I thank the regional, district, and village medical staff Dr. Samwel S. Ulomi, Mrs. Kaale, Dr. Semaruno, Mrs. Valleria H. Mlay, Mrs. Shayo, Dr. Mashafi, UMATI Moshi, Mrs. Margaret Mshana, and the members of KIWAKUKKI.

The ideas in this book have been shared with many friends and colleagues at various points, intellectual and geographical, in the project. My work in Africa was inspired by my first mentor, Don Gordon, *asante sana*. I thank Catharine Newbury, Julius Nyang'oro, Karen Booth, Amy Tsui, Barbara Hicks, and Craig Calhoun for foundational support. A great and collegial debt is owed to my Tanzanianist comrades Melanie Bielefeld, Stacie Colwell, Tim Kelsall, Stacey Langwick, Claire Mercer, Rona Peligal, and Frances Vavrus. I would also like to thank Deborah Barrrett, Caroline Bledsoe, Betsy Hartmann, Amy Kaler, and Susan Watkins for helpful readings from the feminist population angle. I appreciate the support I have received in Denmark from Holger Bernt Hansen, Peter Gibbon, Lene Hansen,

Christian Lund, Hanne Morgensen, and Fiona Wilson. My greatest debts for this book, public and private, are owed to my partner Stefano Ponte and to our *watoto* Sasha Neema, Arianna May, and Zeno William Ponte.

Parts of chapter six are reprinted from "From the Policies to the Clinics: The Reproductive Health Paradox in Post-Adjustment Health Care." *World Development* (2004) 32(6):923–940 with permission from Elsevier.

1

Introduction

From the Policies to the Clinics

How does "overpopulation" create development problems that can be solved through international donor assistance programs aimed at regulating African women's sexual self-discipline? Processes of international development are contingent upon shared understandings of the problem to be solved, yet these are usually taken for granted and only results are scrutinized for effectiveness. When interventions fail to achieve their stated objectives, "politics" are usually to blame, but they are not held up to any systematic analysis. This book analyzes the politics of the emergence of population as a "problem" and family planning as its "solution." How did African countries that were outspoken advocates of "take care of the people and the population will take care of itself" come to embrace typical family planning policies and neoliberal approaches that value limiting a woman's offspring? How do local women and men interpret the changing population messages in ways that make sense as they try to raise healthy children in a context of economic uncertainty?

Family planning practices in Africa are situated within neoliberal notions of modernity, national policies, and global discourses claiming that population is an obstacle to development. The development project—or assisted, driven modernization—is, in theory, a rational bureaucratic means of harnessing, marketing, profiting, and selectively redistributing resources. In practice, it is also a meaning-making project that attributes value through measurement and indicators. Since the Second World War, the point of legitimate state intervention into the intimate and reproductive lives of its citizens has been through population policy. Controlled fertility signifies "modern," predictable,

Westernized relations between the individual body and the body politic. In African countries, the technologies and practices of family planning are promoted as essential gestures for the performance of neoliberal modernity. This book charts how a seamless global population discourse is created through jagged iterations of local practice. How do global discourses like the overpopulation problem get interpreted as they travel from international conferences to policies and clinics? This book answers the question by looking at the effects of international donor discourses on development interventions relying on expatriate, state, and local translators. Three narratives—demographic, development, and feminist—compete for discursive and material precedence. A discourse is not geographically neutral, but is always situated in time and space, and this analysis draws on empirical work from Tanzania. My intention is not to adjudicate success or failure of family planning in Tanzania, but to demonstrate the politics of interpreting a global discourse in the quotidian lives of policymakers, clinic service providers, and local men and women. The interpretive gaps described in this book contribute to our understanding of why there continues to be a familiar disconnect between international development, national policies, and local implementation.

Population policies provide a unique realm of inquiry into the power of development. First, they are considered one of the few legitimate grounds for discussions of gender—women were first brought into development through schemes to control their fertility. Second, they are prototypes of a development apparatus—both the problems and the solutions of population are created in Washington (and London, Paris, and New York) and presented to the Third World[1] either directly by Western consultants and donors or indirectly by an effectively trained cadre of "local" experts. Third, population policies are attempts to bring the power of the state into the most intimate spheres of citizens' lives—the bedrooms and the family.

The shifting global population discourse, integration of HIV/AIDS into reproductive health, and the changing value of children are explored in this book as important directions for the future. In fact, reproductive health in many African communities might be best understood as remaining healthy long enough to reproduce. The translational politics portrayed in this book must be understood if the interpretive gaps between global discourses and local development interventions are to become narrower.

While characterizing the population discourse and its effects as global points to a similar logic and apparatus throughout the Third

World, Tanzania provides a particularly revealing example of the peregrinations between global and local. Unlike the notorious examples of state-led coercive birth control, such as China's one-child policy in 1979 or India's forced sterilizations under the Emergency in the mid-1970s, population policy in Tanzania represents a softer version of reproductive control. However, even in this muted variety, certain family resemblances stand out. The global population discourse assumes that it is possible to specify a generic and permanent solution to the "problem" of population for all people in all places.

When an interview respondent in rural Tanzania replies that her children are "enough" [*wanatosha*], how do we begin to categorize this statement? Scott suggests: "there is no single, all-purpose, correct answer to a question involving measurement unless we specify the relevant local concerns that give rise to the question" (1998, 26). When local concerns draw on global constructions of meaning, as they necessarily do in the context of development, we must grapple with the processes of meaning making and not simply with what appear to be their outcomes.

The incontestable "good" of health is embraced by both proponents and critics of development, modernization, and globalization. The attribution of value and the basis for legitimate distinctions made on its behalf come from a *doxa* (Bourdieu 1999) or dominant vision of process and progress. Yet, despite its universal appeal, the meaning of health and its constituent elements crosses rugged terrain from individual psychology to communal belief systems or culture. Reconstituting the relationship between individual and communal relationship and responsibility for health is part of the development project. People become users, clients, consumers, activists, beneficiaries, stakeholders, and patients within a system that is perhaps neither systematic nor bureaucratic, but that shapes the relationship between those who seek and those who provide health care.

There is disagreement even among those nations providing development assistance as to whether health is a privilege to which one may aspire or a right that is juridically guaranteed. Still, the right and responsibility for one's own health is located in a particularly modernist perception of the individual, and reproductive health accountability rests upon a gendered individual. In Western family planning discourses there are politically charged debates over the extent to which the individual woman is responsible for control of her own body's reproduction. An individual, to varying extents autonomous, is assumed to make decisions and thus "control" her sexual behavior, her actions during fetal gestation, and the outcome of her procreative process. While centering reproductive control on the female body seems "natural," there is no necessary link between procreative possibility and reproductive decision making, as both differences in history and geography make clear. "It is also because matters of culture, and in particular the social divisions and hierarchies associated with them, are constituted as such by the actions of the state which, by instituting them both in things and in minds, confers upon the cultural arbitrary all the appearances of the natural" (Bourdieu 1999, 70).

There is nothing natural about blaming African women for global problems of overpopulation. Campaigns to begin bringing men into reproductive decision making and child rearing signify the extent to which women have been left to shoulder both the biological and moral responsibility for pregnancy and its outcome in most societies. This is not to say that the meanings that Tanzanians give to reproduction, children, or family planning are uniform, stilted by Western meanings, or any more "inauthentic" than such meanings given in the Western cultural context. However, the notion of assisted modernization—the development project—is unique in harnessing international financing and global discourses toward local interventions that both intentionally and haphazardly affect local moral discourses of relation and procreation.

Part of the process of modernization of the contemporary development project is to create women as semi-autonomous actors capable of reproductive decision making in their own right, while simultaneously creating a calculus of value that differentiates good choices from bad ones. It does so in ways that are more intimately linked to the wider processes of globalization and economic change than to historical understandings of the meaning of children, child-bearing, and gender relations within society. We cannot understand family planning or contraceptive choice as taking place in isolation from the differing and contested notions of development and modernity.

International politics, national policies, and local prejudices all interact in structuring relationships at local clinics. Tanzanian women as both service providers and clients must negotiate family planning. While these women are pragmatic (see Lock and Kaufert 1998) in their reproductive strategies, their choices are also prearranged by nearby and distant discourses. A development apparatus creates problems, like overpopulation in a way that structures possible solutions (see Ferguson 1994), without determining outcomes (see Cruikshank

1999). Within this discourse, modern contraceptives function as the ultimate "technologies of sex," (Foucault 1980) disciplining bodies through their life-giving powers of emancipating the modern subject (i.e., freeing women and families from the burdens of children).

The very modern technologies that identify service providers as experts also require them to negotiate between the demands of local clients and the family planning expectations that bodies will be the same due to the preconfigured user of each technology. The discourses of modern contraceptives "efface the materiality of the body and the social contexts within which bodies are experienced and constructed" (Brush 1998, 22). When "other" bodies exhibit their differences, it is the service providers who must negotiate and translate between expectations. Reflecting the perceptions of a global population discourse that blames Third World women for overproduction, and perhaps more than a bit of job frustration (see also Allen 2004; Booth 2004), service providers construct their own notions of these undisciplined bodies that are constantly thwarting the providers' best attempts to "modernize" them. Local women in this context of layered and unequal power relations and constructions of their own identity choose to accept or reject modern family planning according to their own perceptions of need. Politics permeate service provision.

The most well-charted narrative in the global population discourse is the demographic narrative that assumes that overpopulation is a fundamental obstacle to development. The second development narrative links improved socioeconomic status to the population challenge. The third and historically most recent narrative is the feminist narrative that assumes that women's empowerment and gender equality are population problems that must be solved in order to achieve development. In Tanzania, interactions between policymakers and international donors more adequately reflect a global population discourse than they do the experiences of local Tanzanian women. This is in part attributable to the resonance between the global discursive understanding of how local women "are" and the biases held by Tanzanians that separate the interests and identities of policymakers and service providers from those of their female clients. More than two years of fieldwork conducted in the local language suggests that the way that family planning itself is created and recreated at all levels of interpretation reproduces the assumptions and values of a global population discourse that has historically been wedded to population-control ideologies. Thus, policies promoted under the contemporary agenda of reproductive health will need to significantly change the ways that these policies are conceptualized and implemented. Such a radical shift would entail the creation of new development subjects and would alter ways of doing development.

States and Statistics: From Population to Political Economy

The literature on population is commonly criticized for asserting a sterile, positivist view of human reproduction in which little is understood about how these processes take place and even less about what they might mean. The blame is put onto this literature's heavy reliance on demography, a policy-oriented, empirical pursuit wedded to the truths created by statistical relevance.

Statistics embody a "quintessential modernist scheme" (Tilly 1999, 338) and population is, in fact, a concept possible only in the statistical sense (see also Duden 1993). The discourses of development, whether academic or applied (Ferguson 1997), deviate very little in the categories used to organize the messy phenomena of human reproduction. We are all, to paraphrase Bourdieu (1999), thinking like states. Calhoun elaborates this argument that "the categories with which states 'think' structure too much of the thinking of all of us in modern society; breaking with them is a struggle but an important one" (2003, 18).

To begin to think about family planning experiences in an un-statelike fashion, we must question the core of the assumptions about population. Scott (1998) quotes a prosaic tale of eighteenth-century-Prussian forestry to illustrate the important critique of diverse standardizing schemes that operate in the interest of isolating and maximizing some single element of instrumental value. In the example, a single, precise, standardized tree (*Normalbaum*) is developed by a collaboration of mathematicians and foresters. While forests of such trees were both manageable and legible by the state, their lack of diversification led to "forest deaths" as the rationalized trees were subjected to less-engineered forces. The Normal Tree holds lessons for the Normal Family. This book examines family planning in Tanzania and the global population discourse and discontent to demonstrate, as described by Tilly, "the impact of top-down imposition of rationalizing schemes on the recalcitrant complexity of local social life" (1999, 332). In doing so, it describes the processes that act as mediating mechanisms between the abstract, centrally promoted plans and small-scale social life.

One of the goals of this book is to argue that family planning does not belong in the realm of personal decision making, individual health, or happenstance, but is one constituent arena of the global political economy. The term "political economy" is used to mean quite different things by diverse constituencies. Anthropologists are now calling for multi-sited ethnography addressing the political economy as a way to link where they come from to the places they study. Economists use the term to designate the nonobjective, and often ideologically driven work done at the margins of mainstream economics. This book uses the global political economy in terms put forth by feminist international relations. Drawing on Peterson (2002), such a political economy comes into existence through the interaction of *reproductive, productive*, and *virtual economies.*

The link between family planning and the reproductive economy is most intuitive. It is within the reproductive economy that negotiations take place over the conditions of biological reproduction of the community.[2] Human reproduction, historically associated with the domestic, the feminine, appears "natural" but is in fact both public and political. Thus family planning is intimately linked to gender negotiations over childbearing, to norms and expectations of mothers, to questions of acceptable risk, inconvenience or side effects, to reproductive "choice," and to the meanings given to children, proper timing, and reproductive morality. The meaning of successful reproduction in countries like Tanzania is being changed: it no longer means caring for an average of seven children, but now means caring for two children, plus wage-earning labor, plus successful birth control.

The productive economy is the one most familiarly termed "economic" and involves "products (objects, services, commodities, property), factors of production (symbolic and material resources, labor), the processes of production, and processes by which goods are consumed. But it also involves identities and the production of desires and tastes" (Ibid., 6). The relationship between family planning and the productive economy is evident in the historical debates over population growth and development, but also at the local level in the content of messages used to promote family planning, the reasons elaborated by those persons who choose to accept it, and the limitations in the family planning environment in poor countries. Women and couples are encouraged to use family planning in order to bear fewer children to reduce the economic strain on the household and increase the investment of resources per child. Family planning users most frequently describe *maisha magumu*—"tough life"—in terms of the costs of education, health care, and clothing as reasons for choosing a smaller family than their parents had. Finally, the productive economy is the basis of the meaning of underdevelopment in Tanzania. Tanzania is a "heavily-indebted poor country," "recipient," "Third World," "resource-poor," "post-conditonality"[3] state because of the character of its productive economy. These economic conditions constrain the kinds of family planning services that are made available to Tanzanians and also shape the motivations for planning families in particular ways.

Finally, it is within the virtual economy of meaning-making that family planning has its most interesting manifestation. Family planning is one of the ways in which market logic is being introduced into cultural life (see Anagnost 2004). In the demographic transition, "family" is taken over by the market, with its distinctions between quantity and quality. Where children may have once constituted a means of noncommodified pleasure, they now should be valued in terms of their potential contributions and burdens on the family unit. Parents (mostly mothers) are persuaded through public health educational campaigns to have fewer children so that they can purchase more goods: better healthcare, education, and an overall higher quality of life for the family—all of which are becoming increasingly expensive. Contraceptives themselves are an important part of meaning-making in the political economy of the sign, and this book will show how these technologies operate as identity artifacts within the clinic context in Tanzania. Taken together, the reproductive, productive, and virtual economies map a material and symbolic context for family planning by individuals and society.

Disciplined Bodies: Gender, Culture, and Family Planning

How did a lack of self-control by African women come to receive the blame for causing underdevelopment in African societies? One of the earliest modern articulations of the role of self-discipline in constructing society was Emile Durkheim. Durkheim had a notion of each person as part individual and part society, and thus each person places internal constraints on behavior in order to maintain the categories of rational thought. Governing the individual within the disciplining categories of the social is necessary for survival. According to

Durkheim (1961 [1915]):

> If men did not agree upon these essential ideas at every moment, if they did not have the same conception of time, space, cause, number, etc., all contact between their minds would be impossible, and with that, all life together. Thus society could not abandon the categories to the free choice of the individual without abandoning itself (Ibid., 30).

Here, there is a strong notion of society as an independent entity with needs that translate into legitimate demands made on the individual. This opens the door for later theorists who depict a grid of disciplinary powers that actually construct the individual. "Discipline 'makes' individuals: it is the specific technique of a power that regards individuals both as objects and as instruments of its exercise" (Foucault 1979, 170). "Discipline in general, like its most rational offspring, bureaucracy, is impersonal. Unfailingly neutral, it places itself at the disposal of every power that claims its service and knows how to promote it" (Weber 1978, 1149).

Nowhere is the link between individually disciplined bodies and national development more explicit than in the discourse of population as it is presented to Third World women. Foucault describes through his notion of bio-power[4] how "this technology of sex was a whole series of different tactics that combined in varying proportions the objective of disciplining the body and that of regulating populations" (Foucault 1980, 146). I would like to suggest modern contraceptives as the ultimate technologies of sex, and the international population discourse as a regulating apparatus that operates in Tanzania constructing, controlling, and regulating bodies. Bio-power emphasizes the productive, creative, and potentially fulfilling aspects of governance. It is a useful representation of the power of development as contrasted to colonial power (Brigg 2002). Bio-power refers to the regime of government placing the transformation of the human life through knowledge-power technologies as the central obligation of the state. Bio-power coalesces around two distinct poles: the human species (as defined by scientific categories such as population, fertility, etc.) and the human body (as an object to be manipulated and controlled) (Rabinow 1984, 17).

Modern family planning as well is meant to be a technology for transforming individuals. In ways analogous to the prison's production of "delinquents" (Foucault 1979), the global population discourse produces "family planners"—those women[5] whose bodies are properly disciplined according to the needs of the neoliberal community. However the presentation of "needs" is framed in the language of individual rights, children's health, and national development when local women are being sensitized to the population problem.

The modern state requires a particular type of modern disciplined bodies. However, Foucault failed to recognize the explicitly gendered nature of associating undisciplined bodies with things premodern, traditional, backward, and feminine. Apffel-Marglin describes how "women presented a particular problem to the onward march of reason. Reason came to be seen in the eighteenth and nineteenth centuries as antithetical to the experiences of menstruation, gestation, birth, and lactation" (1996, 151). Indeed, it is these feminine experiences that most call for control by disciplining practices. Hunt's seminal work (1988, 1999) describes the lengths to which the colonial regime would go to regulate the bodies of Congolese women through the institution of a proper breastfeeding regime coupled with socialization to become good mothers. Their efforts were a response to the "demographic panic of the 1920s." While the maternal "education," feeding, and surveillance mechanisms were linked to a pro-fertility discourse, Hunt links the colonial need to control intimate aspects of African women's lives to the contemporary attempts by family planning experts to appropriate "this ancestral precedent" of abstinence while nursing as a "banner" for programs encouraging the use of modern contraceptives. Similarly, Vaughan (1991) describes how African women were central to the missionary medical concerns of maternal and child health linked to the perception of African women as the repositories of "all that was dark and evil in African culture and social practices" (1991, 23).

Discourses of choice and responsibility in contemporary Tanzania hinge on the existence of a particular type of female body. The disciplined body feminine is necessary to create the modern body politic/economic. The body politic is defined by Lock and Scheper-Hughes as "the regulation, surveillance, and control of bodies (individual and collective) in reproduction and sexuality, work, leisure and sickness" (Lock and Scheper-Hughes 1996, 45). The body economic is linked to the physical body as described by Foucault through the development of bio-power: "this bio-power was, without question, an indispensable element in the development of capitalism; the latter would not have been possible without the controlled insertion of bodies into the machinery of production and the adjustment of the phenomena of population to economic processes" (1980, 140, 141).

Drawing on the work of Mary Douglas (1966), Lock and Scheper-Hughes argue that "when the sense of social order is threatened, boundaries between the individual and political bodies become blurred, and there is a strong concern with matters of ritual and sexual purity, often expressed in vigilance over social and bodily boundaries" (Lock and Scheper-Hughes 1996, 61). I would like to ponder this notion from a different vantage point, one that links global processes with the local realities of Tanzanian women. Perhaps, the sense of social order is threatened on the global level by terrorism, increasing economic instability, the contagion of cultural homogenization, and an environment that will not indefinitely sustain current human lifestyles. Therefore, the response is vigilance at the level of individual women's bodies justified by the popular myth of African women as profligate reproducers breeding their societies into poverty. International perceptions of the chaotic lead to local calls for control.

In this case, the blurring of the individual and political bodily boundaries is centered in the areas of geopolitical weakness, that is, the Third World. The strong concern over sexual purity and vigilance over social and bodily boundaries is seen in the rational, sterile, global population discourse. I am not making the claim that privileged interests in the First World directly and successfully manipulate Tanzanian women's bodies to serve their own ends. Instead, this book shows how the reality is more complex than that. The population discourse itself, constructed by and constructing how we think about population as a problem, limits the ways that we can think of its solution.

Many theorists of discourse discuss the dissemination of ideas and power as something nebulous, indistinct, and shifting (see Foucault 1979). The power of the global population discourse should not be understood as intentional, singular, or "top-down" power. It is the diffuseness of its power, often the absence of overt force, yet the ordering mechanisms of bodily governance (see Brigg 2002) that we see when we look at what discourse does. Drawing on Ferguson's work (1994, 1997, 1999) relating power and African development interventions, this book argues that population is governed by closely analogous or even identical population institutions and that these share a common discourse—including a common pool of expertise embodied in population "experts" and a common definition of the problem using similar vocabulary and acronyms where one might normally expect full words. Some interests in the realm of population have more power and others have less. Those with power have primary responsibility for determining how the discourse is constructed and the channels through which it is dispersed. Therefore, when we are speaking of shifts in the global population discourse, we should remember to associate this with material changes: new topics for international seminars, different terminology for international assistance's strategic objectives, revised protocols and research themes, new institutional forms and links between players in public and private sectors, amended technical guidelines, improved training programs, reworked protocols for service provision, and the movement of resources from one site to another.

Another common pitfall of discourse analysis is a misunderstanding of discourse as narrative to be counterposed against empirical reality or practice. Yet, discourses both constitute and are constituted by reality (see Hansen 2006). Furthermore, in the words of Cruikshank, "social construction is just not that simple or straightforward. The system and its makers do not create order from above; rather, the messiness of small things makes possible a large system" (1999, 42). A challenge of this book is to trace gaps in the discourse on population—to point out what is *not* being said about reproduction in Africa and how what is being said is often compartmentalized, or "ghettoized" so that it does not disrupt development business as usual. The global population discourse is critical for setting up the development problem to be solved, and thus for structuring the parameters of possible solutions. Population policy articulates this discourse.

From Fertility Control to Reproductive Health: Shifting International Agendas

Rethinking population policy forces us to reconsider the politics of inclusion and exclusion, and the dynamics that both reinforce boundaries and limit the movement and self-determination of the excluded in controlling their own reproduction and health. These exclusionary politics are as important to shaping health in the North as in the South (Keysers 1999). Population issues have been central to notions of international development. National population policies throughout the Third World emerged from an international historical regime that defined the meaning of "population" (Barrett and Frank 1999, 199). The history of this population discourse can be traced to the eugenics movement[6] in the second half of the nineteenth century. It has linked the local needs of the poor for family planning with the fears of the rich of global overpopulation. Population control came to be linked with American foreign policy at the end of the Second World War responding to fears created by the Axis powers' use of population pressures (*lebensraum*) as a justification for their expansionist policies. Fertility control of African, Asian, and Latin American women has been linked to the important policy objectives of economic growth, preserving political stability, and environmental sustainability (Bandarage 1997; Chesler 2005; Furedi 1997; Hartmann 1995; Kabeer 1994; Silliman and King 1999).

Demography, with its core conceptual assumption of universal progress toward low fertility (Greenhalgh 1995; Kirk 1996; van de Kaa 1996), gained prominence as a "policy science,"(Hodgson 1983) the handmaiden of the global population discourse. Ideology has always been pivotal in how demography was formed and financed, and in how it has been used to rationalize key demographic agendas (Presser 1997). Then, "the American vision of population studies became the global vision" (Sharpless 1997, 183). Large-scale surveys, financed as part of development assistance, were undertaken throughout the Third World, and their results were used to support the population control agenda with the power of science (Riley and McCarthy 2003).[7] Overpopulation provided the crisis necessary for mobilizing international support and national policies.

The politics of such policies, often concealed under technocratic language and scientific evidence, erupted during the three international population conferences. In 1974, the Bucharest conference challenged demographic population control with Marxist developmentalism. The Soviet Union, the Vatican, and John Rockefeller joined most of the Third World in questioning the necessity of conventional population control (Finkle and Crane 1975). Attended by a vocal and optimistic contingent from newly independent Third World countries, a consensus emerged epitomized by "development is the best contraceptive" and "take care of the people and the population will take care of itself." International population programs and family planning interventions were criticized for their ideological underpinnings of racism, imperialism, and xenophobia. The next international conference in Mexico City saw different alliances but the same issues for debate. The international development context had changed significantly and the optimism of the previous decade was squelched by economic crises in many Third World countries. By 1984, "developing countries were in a different frame of mind. They no longer spoke of international population assistance as racist, genocidal, or imperialistic, or accused Western nations of advocating population control as a substitute for foreign aid" (Finkle and Crane 1985, 1). In fact, by this time, the interplay between the economic crises, financial aid dependency, and neo-Malthusian goals of donors and lenders had led most Third World countries to move toward development and implementation of conformist population policies. Still, as Watkins argues, "fertility declines, if and when they occur, are almost invariably portrayed as resulting entirely from the agency of individual local actors: colonial governments and the World Bank are rarely seen, nor are gossip networks" (2000, 747).

Conventional population policies come from a blueprint based on the universalizing truths of demography and laid over administrative functionalism of international development assistance. In his classic multicountry study of population policy in the Third World, Warwick (1982) outlines the following generic assumptions behind the promotion of family planning programs as the solution to population problems:

- Irrespective of their social, cultural, and economic circumstances, women of reproductive age want to limit their fertility.
- The motivation to limit fertility can be accurately measured through survey research.
- People motivated to limit fertility will take action to carry out their desire.
- People acting to limit fertility will make use of organized family planning services.
- Individuals not motivated to practice family planning can be made interested though information-education-communication (IEC) programs.
- Individuals who once make use of modern family planning methods will continue to use them until they no longer need them.
- In developing population policies, product is more important than process.
- Population policies are best developed by the central government.
- Family planning programs should be mounted with standard parts and uniform methods of assembly.
- In the development and implementation of population policies sociocultural and economic contexts are largely irrelevant.
- Once harnessed to the structures of government, family planning programs can be implemented through the force of top-down authority.
- The paramount need of clients is for modern family planning services; other needs are either secondary or irrelevant (Warwick 1982).

These assumptions are based on demographic truths gleaned from the last half-century of survey research in the Third World, and they reflect the limitations of this knowledge.

Demographers have been successful in translating complex statistical truths into an easily understandable rhetoric for laypeople, including policymakers and their political constituents in the West. Books such as Erlich's *The Population Bomb* (1968) and *The Population Explosion* (1990)[8] gripped the popular imagination and instilled fear of overpopulation as the most urgent threat to Western security. While publications such as these supported a conservative, determinist demographic agenda that overpopulation was *the* problem hindering international development efforts, actual demographic evidence presents contradictory stories (see Furedi 1997). Purveyors of different levels of demographic knowledge, including feminist demographers, women's health activists, Marxist academics, and population policymakers began questioning the strength of the relationship between population and development, its directionality and its implications for policy. These dissenting voices sparked enough debate to loosen the pillars upon which Third World countries had for decades been told to base their population policies.

A strong push by women's health activists at the 1994 Cairo Conference reflected critically on policies based on fertility control instead of reproductive rights (see Hodgson and Watkins 1997; Sinding and Caldwell 1997; Jain 1998). As elaborated by the United Nations Population Fund, "reproductive health is a positive state, not merely the absence of disease or infirmity…[It] exists in a broader context…[that] includes action towards gender equity, including equal access for women to health care and education, income-generating opportunities, and work in the professional, academic and political spheres" (United Nations Population Fund 1994d, 31). This broad interpretation of reproductive health was expanded to emphasize sexual rights at the 1995 UN Fourth World Conference on Women in Beijing.[9]

> Population and family planning programs should be framed in the context of health and livelihood agendas, give serious consideration to women's health advocates, and be supportive of women's reproductive health and rights. This has to be more than lip service; it requires reorienting international assistance and national policy, reshaping programs, and rethinking research questions and methodologies. Using the language of welfare, gender equity, or health while continuing family planning as usual will not meet the need (Sen 1994, 71).

Hodgson and Watkins (1997) suggest that the Cairo consensus reflected a fragile alliance between American neo-Malthusians and American feminists,[10] locating the discourse firmly in the international arena but arguing that it would be Third World governments, many of which are staffed with American-trained neo-Malthusians, that would shape the implementation of reproductive health. Thus, by the late-1990s, population polices were being renamed and ostensibly revised as "reproductive health" policies framed by a shifting discourse that would link population, health, gender, and development issues. The key words characteristic of development intervention into Third World population issues have shifted as shown in table 1.1.

Table 1.1 Shifting Discourses on Population and Family Planning

Pre-Cairo (1994)	*Post-Cairo*
Neo-Malthusian	Reproductive health
Population control	Empowerment
"Negative"	"Positive"
Individual	Agent
Explicit	Implicit
Conditionality-structural adjustment	Post-conditionality
Stick	Carrot
Trickle-down	Partnership
Demographic, development	Feminist, development, demographic

Source: Original Data.

The movement of concepts from one column to the next has not been comprehensive, simultaneous, or irreversible due to time lag, residual meaning, and memory. However, we will see how these concepts shape the population discourse in practice for the case of Tanzania.

Now, a full decade after the Cairo Declaration, most assessments of international development progress in reproductive health have been disappointing. Third World policymakers "pick and choose" between the aspects of the reproductive health agenda that suit them (Luke and Watkins 2002), as we will see in the Tanzanian case. Furthermore, it is common knowledge that most Western countries have not lived up to the financial commitments made to support the goals of Cairo and Beijing, particularly the United States that has even cut back its funding of sexual and reproductive health programs in the Third World to support the administration's right-wing ideology. In a symbolic, but disturbing move, the American president even refused to reaffirm the Beijing Declaration because it endorses sexual and reproductive healthcare (Chesler 2005, 16). These controversies have demonstrated effects in local provision of reproductive health care around the world (see Knudsen 2006). Conflicts in development interventions and implementation reflect competing discourses of global population.

Discourses and Discontent

The power of language and the power embedded in language are often taken for granted by social scientists, but are well theorized in social theory. Bourdieu explains that "discourses are always to some extent *euphemisms* inspired by the concern to 'speak well,' to 'speak properly,' to produce the products that respond to the demands of a certain market; they are *compromise formations* resulting from a transaction between the expressive interest (what is to be said) and the censorship inherent in particular relations of linguistic production" (Bourdieu 1991, 78, 79). To analyze discourses is to look for framings of meaning and lenses of interpretation, rather than objective, historical truths (see Hansen 2006).

This book examines the global population discourse as a slice from the meta-narrative of neoliberal modernity, and demonstrates how that discourse is constantly being created and recreated through multilayered negotiations. The genealogy of the global population discourse begins when population became a category in which states could begin to conceptualize and thus order their constituents. Simultaneously, population evolved as an area that can be controlled through governance because human reproduction could be controlled by individual restraint. As development was created as a marker for modernity, the global population discourse located population as a site for intervention in promoting the development goal. Thus, population became a problem for development. But what kind of problem is it? In what ways is population a problem? Why is population a problem? What should be done about the population problem? Differing analytical narratives, each with its corresponding practical agenda have held interpretive power over the problem of population at the global and local levels.

There are three global narratives within the realm of population and family planning as shown in table 1.2. The most well-charted narrative in the global population discourse is the demographic narrative that assumes that overpopulation is a fundamental obstacle to development. The second approach is the development narrative that links improved socioeconomic status as the population challenge.

Table 1.2 Narratives of the Population and Family Planning Discourse

Narrative	*Demographic*	*Development*	*Feminist*
Goal	Population decline	Improve economic status	Women's empowerment and gender equality
Interpretive lenses on the population problem and how the state should intervene	"Negative" quantity/numerical	"Positive" quality	"Positive" quality
Advantage	Funding	"Felt need"	International activism
Disadvantage	Links to imperialism, racism, social control	Breadth, expense, complexity	Least visible on the ground, lack of consensus on goals

Source: Original Data.

The third and historically most recent narrative is the feminist narrative that assumes that women's empowerment and gender equality are population problems that must be solved to achieve development.

Each of these narratives can be found in local manifestations of the global discourse in the Tanzanian case. Chapters two and three describe how national policymakers promoted a more holistic, "positive" interpretation of population that focused on quality issues, while international donors and lenders continued to interpret using a minimalist, or "negative" lens of quantity. Chapter four introduces the ramifications of the feminist lens with the other two, as reproductive health is meant to take gender into account in a local family planning project. Chapters five and six document the negotiations between service providers and clients who must make practical sense of the discursive and material constraints of their contexts.

In pragmatic terms, each of the constituent narratives is promoted in the processes of international development through its own vertical bureaucracy, and turf wars exist at all levels of involvement. There is competition for resources from the international donors and lenders depending primarily on trends in development funding, strategies at the international and national levels, and problems that are "in vogue" at any particular moment in development history. The global population discourse has been dominated by the neo-Malthusian demographic narrative since the Second World War, but traces of the development and feminist narratives still exist, often providing alternative agenda to challenge the demographic vision and priorities. In this book, the feminist narrative is lacking from the discussions in chapters two through four, reflecting the historicity of the discourse and the lack of involvement of Tanzanian women's organizations in formulating population policy or implementing family planning. However, while the global population discourse is continuously being reconstituted by shifts in demographic, development, and feminist agenda, it remains a comprehensive discursive structure, intelligible because of its links to the meta-narrative of neoliberal modernity as the goal for development.

How to be a modern family or how to be a modern state involves questions of governmentality from individual restraint to national discretion. The creation of value and evaluation of quality in a numeric, juridical, "negative," and individualistic way is part and parcel of the discourse on neoliberal modernity. Jurgen Habermas, among others, has reminded us "the globalization of markets, media and other networks no longer leaves any promising option for nations to opt out of capitalist modernization" (Habermas 2005, 28). While the inevitability of such a *telos* is not a sealed fate in the academic imaginary, it looks increasingly likely when studying development. Certainly neoliberal modernity is the only game in town backed by the capital of international development assistance. As this book demonstrates, planning one's family or controlling aspects of human reproduction may have multiple meanings and differing local histories. Still, modern family planning is intimately linked to the development project itself and cannot be understood in local terms that ignore the globality of contraceptive technologies and the concepts that accompany them.

To some extent, Third World women in Tanzania and elsewhere, both providers and clients, present their own "alternative modernity" (Appadurai 1991), as the multiplicity of their responses fall neither into categories of contest or compliance with expected modernity.[11] Yet, women come to talk about family planning as "modern" in ways that reflect their understandings of tradition and the global logics of population control. "New technologies fall onto older cultural terrains, where women interpret their options in light of prior and contradictory meanings of pregnancy and childbearing" (Rapp 1990, 41). Certain methods, like contraceptive pills and injections, are notorious for stirring up trouble between men and women, between young and old, and between social liberals and conservatives, as Kaler demonstrates in her history of contraception in colonial Zimbabwe (2003). Women, both alone and with their partners, have always intervened in the fertility process, but these practices have not always been linked to an agenda of national development or to solving a global problem.

The global population discourse that was foundational for most countries' population policies was surprisingly consistent for half a century. The adoption of national population policies in the Third World was closely linked to international population discourse on the population problem. The policies adopted were strikingly similar (see Barrett 1995) and reflected a belief that overpopulation was an obstacle to development. The most prominent players in this discourse were demographers (primarily American and American-trained) who identified themselves as nonpartisan "scientists" in spite of their clearly political origins within the eugenics movement and ongoing support of a conservative agenda (Presser 2000). These demographers were extremely influential setting the research agenda and linking research findings with advocacy work for family planning programs (see for example, Sharpless, 1997).[12] The politics of population interventions may vary slightly from one context to another, but the definition of population problems as macro-level concerns around fertility levels vastly limited the scope of "legitimate" research issues, particularly for funding purposes.[13]

As discussed in the previous section, a shift in the official discourse on population came after the 1994 International Conference on Population and Development in Cairo. An international consensus was generated to support changing the goals of population policies from demographic targets and contraceptive goals to improving "women's reproductive health" (see Ashford 2001; Lane 1994), and the Cairo Programme of Action was endorsed by 184 governments, and even, with some significant reservations, by the Holy See that represents the Catholic church at the United Nations (Chesler 2005, 13). Concepts of women's empowerment, reproductive rights, and sexual health had been important in the women's health advocacy movement for more than 15 years before the Cairo conference, but they had made little inroads into the "science" of population analysis (Presser and Sen 2000; Sen and Batliwala 2000).

The processes and outcome of the Cairo conference ignited both official and anecdotal debates. However, it is generally agreed that the old demography guard was blindsided by a well-organized amalgam of Southern and Northern-based women's health advocacy groups who managed to put gender issues and health problems in the place of the long-popular "population bomb."[14] The debates, of course, are over whether or not this was a good thing. Dixon-Mueller and Germain (2000) conclude with the recognition that broadening the definition of population policy from family planning to reproductive health is "challenging from a political perspective" and requires "a process of institutional rethinking, coordination, and reallocation of resources" out of ministries of health and family planning and into the other "development"-oriented ministries. They summarize the barrage of criticism against the reproductive health agenda:

> ICPD [the Cairo conference] represents a political victory for women, these critics acknowledge, but where is the sense of urgency about high rates of population growth that continue to confront governments and societies in many parts of the world? Where are the population projections, the demographic analyses? Where are the goals for contraceptive acceptance and fertility decline? *Where, indeed, is the population policy*? (Dixon-Mueller and Germain 2000, 69, emphasis added).

The sort of negative responses summarized in this quotation reflect ideological differences more than scientific ones (Presser 2000, 401) but nonetheless, the politics of Cairo continue at all levels of implementation.

While diverse organizations from North and South were able to negotiate a strategic consensus at Cairo that produced the appearance of a cultural transformation in relation to reproductive rights across the globe, the challenges of implementing such an all-encompassing agenda have brought attention to the cultural assumptions that underpin such an agreement. Some proponents claim that the broad strategy of reproductive health would be more effective than policies narrowly focusing on women's control of fertility (Sen, Germaine, and Chen 1994). Chesler (2005) emphasizes that this is a point that should not be taken for granted, as it is often misunderstood. "However strong their disagreements with the past practices of often alarmist and heavy-handed population programs—however serious their commitment to programmatic reforms—they did not deny the benefits of effective family planning to the welfare of individuals, families, communities and eventually, entire countries" (Hodgson and Watkins 1997 cited in Chesler 2005, 13). Some critics claim that "the battle won over the reproductive rights agenda based on a human rights and democratic framework fatally pushed to one side the more politically contentious and difficult issues of economic development" (Harcourt 1999, 9). Cairo did not challenge the underlying assumptions of development with its basis premises of economic growth and modernization. The Cairo agenda, as termed by one critic, is "population control with a woman's face within the overall frame of development business as usual" (Keysers 1999, 21).

Another source of criticism of the Cairo "consensus" is that it diffused the support that had been generated to fund the battle against overpopulation. The lost crisis threatened to lessen support to the reproductive health agenda in general, and to the family planning component in particular. For example, the introduction to a book entitled *How and Why Population Matters*, encapsulates this view:

> The Cairo conference was a remarkable success in so far as it produced a broad and deep consensus on needed actions in the field of population and reproductive health. But Sadik [then Executive-Director of the UNFPA] worried that an important underpinning of the strong political and budgetary support for international cooperation in the field of population that had existed since the original World Population Conference in Bucharest in 1974 was missing from Cairo: the macroeconomic rationale.... The Programme of Action *lacked the sense of urgency* of earlier conferences dealing with *rapid population growth*... (Birdsall, Kelley, et al. 2001, preface, emphasis added).

The lack of a sense of urgency may have implications for population policy implementation throughout the Third World, as the presentation of a population crisis has been a useful tool for public policy creation for population issues. In these circumstances, it is vital to remember: "aid is not like rain that falls on whoever happens to be present in a given time and place. Instead it is more like a set of weights placed on the scales of power at the local, regional and national levels" (Boyce 2002, 240). Thus, the critical links between population policy, external expertise, and foreign aid suggest that most of the priorities of local implementation can be understood as responding to the weight of international agendas.

Synopsis of Chapters

This book weds poststructuralist deconstructions of discourse and power together with feminist political economy in a way that elucidates the links between control of the individual body through family planning and control of the modern state through development. Between some chapters, there is an "intermezzo" to provide an ethnographic snapshot of the policy and research context as it was taking place. More than simply amusing stories, these vignettes interrogate functionalist characterizations of the arid bureaucracy of development. Chapter two begins with the historical journey of the creation of African population policies. International politics between states and donors and lenders play an important role in shaping the perceptions of African countries' population "problem" and its possible solutions. The shifting positions of the Tanzanian state are described as strategic ambiguity within the context of its national development. Organizing the chapter historically allows the reader to consider the analysis of population within a national context of negotiating development policies in postcolonial states, as well as within the international context of donor optimism, economic debacle, structural adjustment, and its aftermath. This chapter includes a rich and detailed case study based on internal and external government documents, interviews and participant observation at critical meetings that defined the policy process in Tanzania. Then an intermezzo gives an ethnographic description of the author's day interviewing at the Ministry of Health, including an unplanned encounter between "beltway bandits" and the deputy responsible for family planning.

Chapter three examines the implementation of Tanzania's National Population Policy (NPP) as an exemplary reflection of conflicting population discourses. It looks at the internal struggles over the role of family planning in implementing the policy, the Achilles heel of the entire process. Interviews and external documentation are analyzed through a discursive analysis of power that demonstrates the workings of international and national population politics. Family planning is a policy outcome, historically situated through both government and NGO-based service provision in Tanzania. The roll of the "local" NGO and the coordination of state and non-state actors is important. The chapter argues that the scope of the family planning apparatus has changed significantly between the time of the inception of the National Family Planning Programme and current interventions to promote the expanded agenda of reproductive health. However, the character of these interventions and the mediating mechanisms between global discourse and local women remain consistent. In fact, some of the problems encountered with integrating the non-family planning aspects of the reproductive health agenda are traceable to the ambivalent roots of the program and policy environment. Thus, this chapter holds the foundation for many of the general conclusions in the book.

Chapter four describes an archetypal example of attempting to reconcile the demographic, development and feminist narratives of the global population discourse in the practice of a donor-funded intervention. The reproductive health agenda, like other neo-modernization discourses of development progress, assumes that development, feminist and demographic goals are synergistic. This "all good things go together" assumption is challenged when such wide-ranging projects are implemented in a local context of resource scarcity. To make family planning acceptable in the face of local discontent over perceived population control ideologies, one long-running project linked contraceptive provision with other local development objectives. It shows how attempts to "empower" women became trapped between global expectations of population control and local men's desire to shape the project toward their own needs. In the process a local category of "passive acceptor" is invented to mediate between global and local discourses. The chapter epilogue details a field visit with the project's international donors and the performance of global and local in this piece of development theatre.

Chapter five explores the ways that the "modern" family planning interventions construct women themselves within discourses of "tradition" and "modernity." Family planning technologies, more than simply a means for preventing conception, are involved as identity artifacts in the construction of bodies and in the reproduction of power relations. As such, modern contraceptives, organized by and implemented through, donor-funded programs constitute a discursive apparatus through which scattered hegemonies are disseminated. New technologies have been interpreted through existing lenses of traditional family planning strategies. However, tradition itself is being brokered through the needs of legitimacy and modernity, as described earlier in the chapter as "lost knowledge." The entire dichotomy of "traditional" and "modern" constructed at other levels of the discourse on family planning did not make sense in the lives of Tanzanian women themselves. Material conditions in local clinics and in the lives of those who staff them intertwine with markers of identity; thus, family planning provides opportunities for enhancing material and symbolic capital at many levels. Service providers are caught between the prerequisites of modernity including higher contraceptive rates and the realities of dilapidated local clinics and uncooperative local bodies. The chapter epilogue describes the author's attempts at negotiating the health system to get basic health care for a child in a government regional hospital.

Chapter six examines how the recipients of the population discourse, local women, and to some extent their partners, respond to the messages that they are receiving. The chapter argues that there is a generalizable "local lens" for understanding family planning: in countries like Tanzania, family planning focuses on having children, not on avoiding them. In such cultures of childbearing, where deciding to opt out of having children is not really an option for women, the most important thing a contraceptive can do is to enable them to have healthy, well-provided for children. Using comparative work from The Gambia, the chapter argues that the conditions under which a pregnancy becomes auspicious are conditioned by discourses on gender, health, and modernity. The ubiquity of childbearing for adult women, the centrality of maintaining the health of the mother and her children, and the imperative to care for the children properly all shape the context of fertility decision making. These lenses also have implications for how various fertility technologies are perceived and used. Ongoing research in Tanzania suggests that some women and their husbands may be using contraception to have fewer children while others use it to have more. However, the dynamics involved in planning one's family and choosing to use contraception look similar and are likely to exist throughout African high-fertility countries. A concluding intermezzo presents field notes from a revisit to a regional hospital in Tanzania describing the local experiences with decentralization, ongoing but unpredictable donor support, and negotiating the AIDS epidemic and its treatment.

The final chapter draws some conclusions on the local meanings of population, family planning, and development interventions in the context where reproductive health is best understood as remaining healthy enough to reproduce. Global discourses on population have material and symbolic effects on local politics, service provision, and reproductive decision making. The effects of such discourses can be seen in the narratives between donors and the state, between service providers and their clients, and between husbands and wives. Meanings are negotiated, deals are struck, and families are planned within a global discourse, yet everyone is local somewhere. Not surprisingly, discontent emerges at the interface of such a predetermined, static, and homogeneous solution to complex and contingent local problems. In Tanzania, fertility is negotiated within a context shaped by childbearing as an integral part of gender identity, the potential threat posed by untimely pregnancy for both the mother and the existing children, and the modern notion of caring properly for one's family. Family planning is promoted and interpreted as a part of responsible parenthood, not as an alternative to it. Contemporary family planning services must be provided under the rubric of reproductive health, within a context of health care decentralization, and must include HIV/AIDS.

2

Strategic Ambiguity: The Historical Context of the Tanzanian National Population Policy

The time element is important—bring the population growth to zero as quickly as possible. Donors think this is urgent and government should be more active and quick—Tanzanian government official involved in the Population Policy.[1]

Introduction

Every policy has a history, and population policies are state interventions into some of the most intimate and private aspects of citizens' lives. Given the cultural value placed on fertility and lineage and Africa's historical depopulation through slavery, genocide, and famine, population policy is risky business for any African state. Tanzania was one of the first countries in sub-Saharan Africa to begin offering contraceptive services in 1959, yet has been one of the last to declare an official population policy in 1992. Interestingly, Tanzania was also one of the most outspoken Third World countries promoting the idea that population was not a major problem for development at the 1974 World Population Conference in Bucharest. However, when Tanzania adopted a National Population Policy, it looked strikingly similar to those of other Third World countries. As a statement to the international community, the policy signified an important shift in the way the Tanzanian state was approaching its population problem. Given Tanzania's reluctance to declare an official population policy that defined its population as a problem, why did the government finally agree to do so in 1992?

Often, the tangible processes of policymaking in Third World countries are left unexamined as analysis focuses on policy content. Yet, the quotidian grind of policymaking affects both the outcome of the document and the relationships between the actors involved in writing the policy and those meant to implement it. In the official history, Tanzania's National Population Policy was a national response to local needs. The policy resulted from a "growing appreciation in the country of the implications of rapid population growth for the provision of social services and deterioration of natural resources hence, the need to influence population trends both quantitatively and qualitatively using a population policy" (United Republic of Tanzania 1994, 6). The Tanzanian state is portrayed as the dominant force in bringing forward a policy, even though its steps toward such a result were clearly led by international donors.

This chapter traces the global discourse of overpopulation and its interplay with national politics. International donors and national policymakers dominate the scene, and the meanings they give to population issues will shape both understandings and interventions in local clinics. In the early stages of Tanzania's independent political history, the state defined its population problems as those of migration from rural to urban areas and provision of services by the government, particularly in education and health. The Tanzanian government was reluctant to separate out issues of population from a holistic approach to development that focused broadly on poverty. However, during the 1970s and 1980s, explicit debates were ongoing over the scope and direction of population interventions and the possibility or need for a policy.

Over time, the Tanzanian state's approach to population has gradually shifted to become more compatible with the priorities and understandings promoted by its donors and lenders. The most prominent actors in the international population arena are the United States Agency for International Development (USAID), the United Nations Population Fund (UNFPA), the International Planned Parenthood Federation (IPPF) and the Population Council. Historically, the Tanzanian government has maintained a strategically ambiguous stance in its declarations and approaches to population (Richey 1999). This ambiguity exists in both the document of the National Population Policy itself and in the directives promoted by the state for its implementation. Nonetheless, the aspect of the population policy that is, in effect, given the most priority is family planning. This organization of a family planning program as the main or only implementing arm of population policy related to fertility reduction is typical in population policy implementation (Jain 1998). The family planning sector is most visible because it receives the most attention and funding from international donors, the critical sources of development interventions in a time when state-funded health care is rapidly declining in both quantity and quality. Kiondo (1995) began documenting the ongoing process of "donorisation" of important social services as one of the main forms of development privatization taking place in contemporary Tanzania. The donors' emphasis on family planning stems from the way that population is understood as a "problem" in a global discourse that emphasizes reducing fertility levels as a prerequisite to development. Such a demographic emphasis is no longer explicit in the post-Cairo agenda, but the narrative of overpopulation and a desire for fertility reduction remains a the driving force for many interventions. It could be argued that the Tanzanian state, weakened by its dependence on international aid and loans and the conditionalities accompanying its structural adjustment programs, has become even more receptive over time to the agenda of its international donors and lenders in tackling many development issues, including population.

Technically speaking, a population policy is any policy that deals with fertility, mortality, or migration of populations. However, in practice, population policy has been associated with family planning interventions to the point that the two cannot be disentangled from each other. Most informants representing the Tanzanian state claim that family planning is only a small part of the population policy scope, and they try to delink the common association that population policy *means* family planning support. In contrast, supporters of family planning interventions sometimes object to linking a "technical" issue like health care service provision with the "political" debates surrounding the national population policy. Defining the scope and meaning of population policy has been an exercise in politics involving national and international actors situated within a global discourse of overpopulation.

Population must be made a problem because it is usually regarded as simply "politics-as usual" in the realm of policymaking. Thomas and Grindle (1994) draw comparisons across 16 countries, and show that population policy advocates typically tried to convince decision makers that population growth constituted a "crisis." Policy elites play an important role in timing of the policy, shaping the terms of policy debate, and generating consensus on the need for policy change. Population policy reform is generally slow, involves incremental change, includes very little public discussion, is dominated by experts and technical analyses of the population problem, and is critically linked to countries' dependence on continuing good relationships with international donors. This chapter elaborates how demographic, development, and feminist global narratives are integrated, adopted, and adapted in the context of Tanzanian policy.

There are two quite different versions of the history of the population policy as it is summarized in government and donor documents. One cites the introduction of family planning services in the country in 1959 as the first important move in dealing with population issues. The other refers instead to the independent government's censuses conducted since 1967[2] as the marker of official attention to population. One government informant explained: "I'm sure you will get different answers when you ask people what they think the policy is about."[3] This chapter is a discussion of just what the policy is about to show how the problematization of population shaped both the discourses and practices of implementation.

Historically, family planning and population issues were met with resistance in both the political and the popular realms. While it may appear that the Tanzanian government's positions on population and family planning have been oscillating, and at times even contradictory, I argue that the stance has been similar and strategically ambiguous from independence to the present. The dominant discourse about Tanzania's population problem has changed over time reflecting variations in the global discourse on population and reproductive health, but implementation of the policy suggests that while the discourse has shifted, the debates remain.

The realm of population discourse in Tanzania, like politics itself, is full of ambiguity, ambivalence, and strategizing by all actors involved. To disentangle the discursive statements, this chapter will stick closely to texts as spoken or written, often including direct quotations or translations to draw attention to the nuances and stylistic shuffling as the global discourse of overpopulation took precedence in Tanzanian policy circles. Following a timeline of the events in the population policy history, this chapter begins with a discussion of the perceptions of the Tanzanian government from independence until the early 1980s. During this time, population was not considered to be a problem, yet the government enacted implicit population policies. Then the chapter moves into the situation in the 1980s when ideologies were changing in many areas, and population was being redefined and problematized in a particular way. This discussion elaborates on the role of donors and international financial institutions in constructing Tanzania's population problem, and discusses the seminars that were held to build consensus over the need for a policy. The final section draws conclusions, suggesting which issues we can expect to dominate implementation in the future.

Perspectives from the Early Independence Period (1961–1980)

> Tanzania's population problem is not one of absolute numbers or density, but rather the rate at which the population is growing in relation to the country's capacity to meet people's basic needs (United Nations Population Fund 1994b, 7).

Population is Not a Problem

In newly independent Tanzania, donors and development organizations claimed that the government was not aware of the link between population and development. However, documentation from this period shows that government was actually aware of population issues, which it defined largely in relation to other development issues. Yet, the solutions considered desirable by the government for dealing with this issue were not the ones promoted by Tanzania's development organizations and donors. Some of these actors used the rhetoric of clarifying the problem to instead propose a different array of solutions.

Mainland Tanzania has a total documented population of nearly 34 million people in an area of 881,289 square kilometers, or a population density of 38 persons per square kilometer (Census 2002, table 2). As of July 2006, the estimated population rose to over 37 million and it is projected to reach over 59 million by 2025. Still, when compared with most of the Third World, Tanzania is neither a very densely populated nor a highly populous country, yet population has been singled out by donors as a major development problem. The Tanzanian government has not historically viewed its population numbers as a problem. The problem of population in the strictly numerical sense of too many people per square kilometer is legitimate for only a few areas of the country such as Kilimanjaro and Mwanza Regions, but not for the country as a whole. Therefore, unlike other African countries where overall population density is great, population must be problematized in a different way in Tanzania.

During the early independence phase,[4] the Tanzanian government had defined its population problem as migration from rural to urban areas and provision of services by the government, particularly in the fields of education and health. The policy solutions to these problems were implementation of Universal Primary Education (UPE), villagization, and primary health care. Therefore, the government at this time did recognize a link between population and development issues albeit in a different way.

After the colonial period when population growth was clearly seen as a necessary component of economic development, there was some debate over both what the population actually was doing and what it should do. Caldwell (1968) reported that the independent government position was in favor of a larger population and that the birth rate should be higher (Thomas 1979, 12). The United Nations conducted a study of the demographic situation in Tanganyika in 1949, and recommended that a more rapid increase in population was needed (Mkini 1980, 65). Both the colonial and early independence governments followed these pro-natalist recommendations while also noting the need for population redistribution from areas of high density to those of low density.

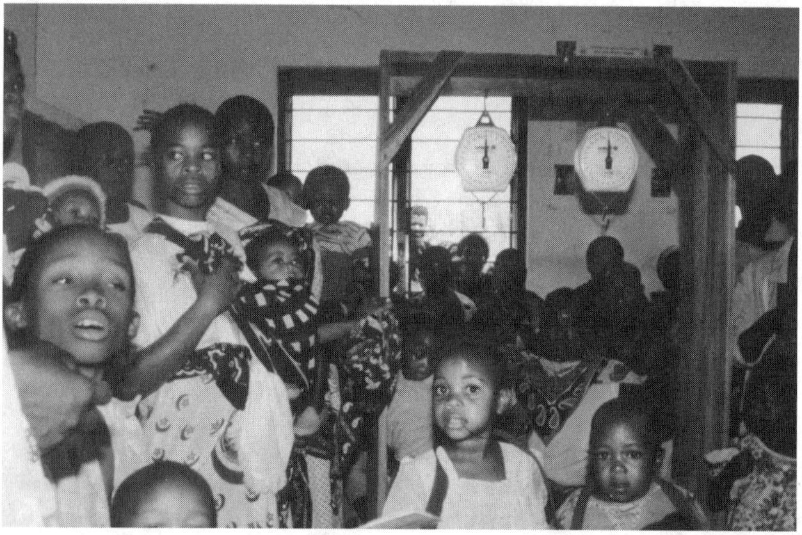

Photo 1 Mothers Wait to Weigh their Children in the Clinic
Source: Photograph by Lisa Ann Richey.

Nyerere's Perspective

In 1969, while presenting the Second Five Year Development Plan to the Annual General Meeting of TANU, then President Nyerere made the statement that was to become the most well-known expression of early government views on population. Nyerere explicitly recognized the link between population and development, yet fertility reduction and family planning were not seen as synonymous with population, nor were they put forth as its solution. After a discussion of the importance of primary school education, Nyerere made reference to the results of the 1967 census that showed the population as more numerous and faster growing than had been previously understood. These new facts set the stage for his often quoted statement about population growth being good, but associated with the responsibility of providing for the increasing numbers of children:

> It is very good to increase our population, because our country is large and there is plenty of unused land. But it is necessary to remember that these 350,000 extra people every year will be babies in arms not workers. They will have to be fed, clothed, given medical attention, schooling, and many other services for very many years before they will be able to contribute to the economy of the country through their work. This is right and proper and is in accordance with the teachings of the Arusha Declaration. But it is obvious that just as the number of our children is increasing, so the burden on the adults—the workers—is also increasing. Giving birth is something in which mankind and animals are equal, but rearing the young, and especially educating them for many years is something which is a unique gift and responsibility of men. It is for this reason that it is important for human beings to put emphasis on caring for children and the ability to look after them properly, rather than thinking about only the numbers of children and the ability to give birth. For it often happens that men's [*sic*] ability to give birth is greater than their ability to bring up the children in a proper manner (Nyerere 1973, 1987, 1988).

In this speech, Nyerere said that it is good to *increase* the population, as had been recommended by earlier consultant missions and the colonial government. Also, people are considered a viable resource for contributing to the economy of their country through their work. Nyerere also said that it is as important to care for children properly, as to give birth to them. However, he did not say that since Tanzanians could not care for their children, they should stop having them. From this perspective, a family with three poorly cared for children is not necessarily any better off than a family with ten similarly impoverished children.

Political support is often believed to be one of the most significant policy factors in determining the success of family planning programs—even more so in countries like Tanzania where the social setting is less favorable (USAID 1979). The lack of political support from African leaders is thought to be an important constraining factor in the implementation of family planning programs on the continent (Azefor 1988; Sai 1988). Political support may be claimed on the basis of explicit statements by leaders or the existence of a national policy, or it may be implicit through what the government actually does—such as creating a favorable legal/regulatory environment or providing adequate resources (Knowles, Bollen, and Yount 1994, 13). The second half of Nyerere's famous quote has been used to claim official political support for family planning in Tanzania before the country developed a population policy.

The Tanzanian family planning association UMATI appropriated Nyerere's speech as a show of support for their own work. UMATI described this quote as a "strong statement advocating for childspacing…a moral booster to UMATI because the Association was still working under difficult conditions with strong opposition and without support from the government" (Mpangile 1994, 8). Indeed, wavering between emphasis on a robust population and pointing to Malthusian relationships between population growth and development will continue around the population policy.

Nyerere's speech was named by many of my informants as a direction-setting moment from the perspective of the Tanzanian government's approach to population. One member of the Population Planning Unit (PPU) referred to Nyerere's speech during an interview to give credibility to the stance taken by the Tanzanian government vis-à-vis international donors:

> It's not easy to say why, but I feel that first of all, the population programs in Tanzania, to some extent, are donor dominated. For example, since independence, the government has been interested in population in one way or another, particularly in the impact of population growth on resources and efforts of the government to [provide for] increasing populations, particularly in the area of social services. For that reason, censuses have been emphasized for evaluating population and defining problems. For example, in the second 5-year development plan, again at the party conference, Nyerere, as president and chair submitted the plan and gave a speech, and among other areas, he talked about the impact of population growth. He gave the famous statement on how easy it is to have children, but it takes time before they are self reliant…the government didn't come up with clear programs to do something about population growth…they had the idea that

> development would make people realize it on their own...(Interview 95GD01b, August 13, 1995).

From this statement, the Nyerere quote is meant to show how the independent Tanzanian government had concerned itself more with development and less with a demographic agenda.

Population issues were politically contentious at home and abroad during the early independence period. The 1974 World Population Conference in Bucharest was marked by an ideological divide between the West and the Third World over disparities in the international economic order and the link between population problems and development (see Finkle and Crane 1975). Tanzania was one of the most vocal Third World delegates—insisting that the focus of the conference should be on the development problem instead of the population problem. "The head of the Tanzanian delegation noted that almost all countries in Africa had suffered severely from colonialism and slavery, hence this experience had taught the African countries that '... for us, people, population are a development asset, the present history of continuing decolonisation is a great testimony of this...the creative and over abundant power of the people to surmount all obstacles'" (Mkini 1980, 64).

Tanzania clarified to the international community its official position in response to the 1976 Third UN Inquiry among governments that its rate of population growth was considered beneficial because it "contributes positively to economic and social development by permitting conservation of environment for future use by providing sufficient population for: environmental maintenance, economic exploitation of natural resources including food production, supply of manpower for economic expansion...[and provides] demographic dynamism sufficient to maintain national innovative capacity, achieve desired levels of replacement of population and to support a national and cultural identity" (United Nations Population Fund 1979, 21). The government also stated that "the present rate of fertility contributed positively to family well-being by making possible achievement of the desired number of children, providing support for aging parents, ensuring continuity (descendancy) of the family, and providing sufficient family labour" (Ibid., 22). In this response, the government was documenting its stance from Bucharest that development, not population growth, was the major problem facing the country. Its solutions were following along with the "take care of the people and the population will take care of itself" ideology.

Institutionalizing Population and Development Issues

Tanzania at the time was "well-known for its attempt to define and follow an independent line of development, aware of its place in the Third World and in Africa, sensitive to the nature of its relations with industrialized nations and aid-donors, and conscious of its distinctive approach to development" (Thomas 1979, 3). Yet, while the Tanzanian state as spokesman for the Third World was maintaining that it had no population problem, it was also considering the links and causal relationships between population and economic growth. One government informant suggested that the newly available census data were causing the government to consider issues of population differently. He said that at Bucharest, "even Mwalimu [Nyerere] did not admit that there was a problem, but when the 1978 census results came out, they realized that the population was growing faster than they had thought."[5] In response to the Bucharest Population Conference resolution calling on governments to appoint demographic staff to advise the government on population issues, the government transferred an unnamed "young demographer" from the Bureau of Statistics to the Development Planning section of the Ministry of Finance and Development Planning in February 1978 (Thomas 1979). This began the institutionalization of population issues in the government. Population issues took on a sense of local controversy. A local news article described how "pressure for a population policy began soon after the 1978 census but when the Government established the Family Planning Association of Tanzania (UMATI), a political rumpus broke out. Some parliamentarians accused government of attempting to prevent births when there were still vast areas of open land to accommodate more people" (Lenga 1987).

Donors began funding seminars to provide the government with an opportunity to discuss the population issue. In October 1974, a seminar was held in Tanga Region organized by the International Labor Organization (ILO) in collaboration with the Tanzanian government and funded by UNFPA. The emphasis of this seminar was "the importance of stimulating widespread consciousness on the positive contribution by trade unions through worker's education in the field of population and economic and social development" (Malima 1980, 169). A more-or-less similar seminar (as characterized by its opening speaker) was held in Arusha Region in 1980. In his introductory speech, Minister Malima noted "As you very well know, we in

Tanzania do not have a population problem as such" (Malima 1980, 170). He went on to explain that despite the unproblematic population density, if the government was to achieve its objectives of socialism and self-reliance, it would be easier to provide for the material well-being of the people with a slowly growing population, rather than a rapidly growing one. The speeches and papers given at this conference dealt with population issues in terms of collecting appropriate demographic data that could then be used to provide services. Little or no mention was made of demographic goals, fertility reduction, or family planning.

Tanzania's Implicit Population Policy

A 1978 paper states that Tanzania already had an implicit population policy based on government "statements, strategies, regulations and legislation all relating to the control and management of population" (Thomas 1979, 1). Drawing on Dye's (1972) models of policy formation, Thomas argued that Tanzania's population policy is best represented by the "group model" where conflicting groups with different interests form the basis for policymaking. Groups active in Tanzania's colonial and earliest independence period were metropolitan governments, local administrations, settler organizations, commercial enterprises, and missionary societies. These organizations stand in contrast to the ones whose influence in population issues began to rise in the late 1970s: external agencies (such as the IPPF, the World Bank, UNDP, USAID), multinational corporations, academic institutions and research bodies, indigenous elites, the political party, the trade unions, and, increasingly, popular opinion (Thomas 1979, 7). Thomas's assertion that Tanzania did indeed have an implicit population policy, in the early independence period makes sense if we consider, as he did, the policies put in place by the government to deal with what it considered to be its problems. However, government policies on primary education and resettlement were not sufficient to convince the international donors that the problem of population was being adequately addressed.

UNFPA documents state "Tanzania has deliberately eschewed adopting an explicit population policy. The Mission fully recognizes this and has no intention of recommending otherwise" (United Nations Population Fund 1979, 88). Donors at the time were aware of the controversy surrounding population control and had to tread carefully to insure that their interventions were not interpreted as coercion. This negotiation involved the creation of a "need" that was left unmet. A study of UNFPA's first Needs Assessment provides a striking example. The document stated that "Tanzania can be characterized as having an implicit population policy" represented by its various policies such as villagization, UPE, and preventive health care, but it went on to qualify that "an appreciation for the impact of these policies on *demographic trends* and the necessity to take them into consideration in planning was expressed...only at a very high level in Government" (United Nations Population Fund 1979, 20, 21, emphasis added).

UNFPA recognized the Tanzanian state's ambiguous stance as "in part deliberate since there was a widespread reluctance to single out population as a topic divorced from the whole gamut of social and economic policies and programmes" (United Nations Population Fund 1979, 21). The Tanzanian state presented its views as a more holistic perspective on population and development. However, UNFPA interpreted this reluctance as resulting from a misunderstanding.[6] UNFPA claimed that Tanzania was unwilling to confront population issues, which consist of more than just fertility regulation. Yet, UNFPA also said that what the Tanzanian government was doing about population issues outside of fertility regulation was insufficient, thus creating the need for development assistance.

In sum, UNFPA's Needs Assessment gave contradictory images of the Tanzanian government. First, the government was described as having an implicit population policy on the basis of its larger social reforms. However, it was criticized for not having an "appreciation for the impact of these policies on demographic trends" and for being "reluctant" to single out population. Then, finally, UNFPA claimed that the Tanzanian government did not want to isolate and deal with the population problem because it was misinformed, believing that population was solely concerned with fertility regulation. However, if the government was dealing with the larger issues that reach beyond fertility regulation, but was still not dealing sufficiently with its population problem according to UNFPA, then the only aspect left unresolved was fertility regulation. Therefore, despite claims to the contrary, the evidence suggests that UNFPA was trying to change the Tanzanian government's perception of population to focus explicitly on fertility control.

At the same time that UNFPA was criticizing the government for its lack of awareness of demographic perspectives, the report tried to argue that antinatalist policies were already being enacted by the Tanzanian state. For example, the Needs Assessment states "In the recent budget speech the provision was made that 'for a person with children there will also be a refund of tax calculated at the rate of Tsh 10 per child per month, up to a maximum of four children.' This seems to suggest an attempt to discourage large families and may thus be classified as an anti-natalist policy" (United Nations Population Fund 1979, 24). UNFPA opined in one section that the government was not willing to single out population because of its "erroneous" linkage with family planning and fertility reduction. Yet, in the same report, UNFPA also claimed that the government really wanted fertility reduction as shown in its antinatalist policy. Despite its continuing claim that the Tanzanian government must be convinced that a population policy is not simply fertility reduction, when trying to find evidence of existing implicit population policies, UNFPA pointed exactly to those policies read as directed toward fertility reduction. Interestingly, despite Tanzania's supposed "antinatalist policy, the Needs Assessment concluded that "in the present Tanzanian context, it would be inappropriate or untimely to recommend the establishment of any special institutional arrangements to formulate, monitor and implement population policy...The Mission therefore recommends that emphasis be placed on changing perceptions rather than defining a population policy" (United Nations Population Fund 1979, 27). As we will see in the following discussion, changing perceptions involves indigenizing the global population discourse, and in doing so, it creates policy.

In sum, donors needed to show that the Tanzanian state actually wanted to do something about its population problem in ways that would fit with the programmatic realities of international assistance. Thus, the Needs Assessment gave evidence of implicit population policies, while arguing that the government was not able to address these issues adequately; therefore, intervention was needed. This intervention should first change the perceptions of the Tanzanian government toward its problems and then devise an explicit policy that represented these changed perceptions. There was no need to push for a policy based on the existing government perceptions—policies of villagization, UPE, and primary health care were already in place.

Seminars to Encourage Awareness of Population

It should be stated quite categorically that UNFPA responds only to the needs of governments as they themselves perceive them and that it does not seek to advocate any particular population policy (Lewis-Jones 1980, 188).

Education became the tool for reconciling between state ideology and international organizations' population interventions. Seminars were recommended for disseminating results from the 1978 census to be used in planning at the national, regional, and local levels. UNFPA stated that "at these seminars, it will be important to discuss the different elements that constitute a population policy as perceived in the Tanzanian context, with the objective of encouraging awareness of population as a comprehensive set of processes affecting all facets of development policy" (United Nations Population Fund 1979, 89). However, the intervention provided was to encourage awareness in the areas where it did not already exist in sufficient concentration: fertility limitation through family planning.

However, because family planning was not one of the policy measures chosen by the Tanzanian government to combat its problems, UNFPA had to claim that family planning was *not* part of its agenda. In a speech at the 1980 National Seminar on Population and Development, the UNFPA coordinator stated:

> Because UNFPA works in a relatively sensitive and in some respects still controversial area, its aims can easily be misunderstood... Where governments have requested help in laying the groundwork for a population policy, we have responded. We also see it as our mandate to promote awareness among policy makers about population issues. Similarly, *family planning programmes* supported by UNFPA are *a response to the priorities expressed by certain governments*, particularly in Asia, where very fast population growth rates have been perceived as a constraint to development. However, and this is particularly true in Africa, in the health sector UNFPA has primarily been concerned with child spacing in the overall context of maternal and child health...In some instances, African countries have also been concerned at their low fertility rates and here UNFPA has responded in several countries with studies and strategies to deal with the problems of infertility and subfecundity (Lewis-Jones 1980, 188, emphasis added).

The quotation emphasizes that, whatever it might have been doing in other parts of the Third World as was well-known through the Bucharest debates, Tanzanians should not be alarmed that UNFPA might advocate a particular population policy focusing on family planning for *them*. The UNFPA representative also noted that "narrower definitions of population...have caused controversy in many countries, including the United Republic of Tanzania" (Viederman 1980, 194). UNFPA tried to define the problem of population in a way that would convert the Tanzanian officials:

> The third myth that is widely believed, without much examination, is that population programmes should be regarded exclusively as family planning programmes. Obviously, this is rooted in the belief that the only population problem one faces is the problem of over-population, which could be tackled by curbing population growth. In fact, population problems and programmes cover a wide range of issues, such as size, growth, distribution, composition, structure, mortality, fertility, migration and many other variables (Viederman 1980, 192).

In the previous statements we can see UNFPA trying strategically to position its objectives with, not against, those of the Tanzanian state. In what comes across as a defensive tone, UNFPA notes that its family planning programs were only a response to the priorities expressed by certain governments. Of course, this must be read in the context of the previously described objectives of changing the way the government thinks about population issues and aligning priorities with an international agenda.

The struggle to define the Tanzanian population discourse continued and further sensitization events were held. Another seminar, entitled The Second African Population Conference was held in Arusha in 1984. The inaugural address given by the Minister of State for Planning and Economic Affairs clarified that "the population problem facing many African countries was essentially a problem of socio-economic development" (United Nations Economic Commission for Africa 1984, 1). He went on to spell out that "Tanzania viewed the Conference as a development planning Conference with emphasis on population rather than a Population Conference per se"(Ibid.). His speech explicitly laid out the state's priorities—"data collection, urbanization and educational progress through economic and social planning"—in contrast to family planning, which was deemed "a controversial issue." Whether or not family planning would be given a role in population efforts was dependent on the donors' ability to come up with the money, and to put it in an area of intervention approved of by the government. In the minister's words, "The pace at which significant family planning efforts would be realized would largely depend on available resources and recognition of the importance of women's education" (United Nations Economic Commission for Africa 1984, 1).

Education, child mortality, infertility, and cultural appropriateness are the pillars of the population policy recommended by the Tanzanian government through the mid-1980s. The government's stance on population was not well-received by international or local proponents of family planning. For example, one article argued: "a serious cause for concern in Tanzania is the fact that people are not prepared to discuss the menacing growth of population due to a false sense of shame" (Worrall 1983). A representative from UMATI describes the 1980s: "there are . . . no indications that the Government is fully aware of the implications of rapid population growth for implementation of national programmes of social and economic development. In fact, the Government is known to have no intentions of instituting any direct policy of reducing the natural increase" (Mkini 1980, 64). Similarly, a WHO representative in Dar es Salaam stated that "the government of the United Republic of Tanzania has not taken any rigid position on population-related issues, neither has it endorsed any overt population control program" (Akerele 1985, 65, 66).

The debate over whether or not the Tanzanian government was actually doing anything about population in the policy realm was shaped more significantly by the needs and goals of the evaluating institutions than by what the government actually was saying or doing at the time. Indeed, the policies implemented by the government in the areas of social service provision and migration could be read as constituting an implicit population policy. However, the existence of an implicit policy of this sort did not require the state's embrace of a population problem. The apparent confusion over whether or not Tanzania actually had a national population policy, long before adoption of the National Population Policy in 1992, can be clarified by recognizing the dual usage of the term "population policy" within the discourse of the population problem. First, there was agreement on an implicit population policy as found in statements by representatives from the government, donors, and academic consultants. However, these implicit policies were not the ones being promoted by international donors as necessary for dealing with population issues in the country, and only proper recognition of such a problem would lead to adoption and implementation of the right kind of explicit population policy.

The 1980s: Geopolitics, Ideology, and Shifting Ground

Throughout the 1980s, changes began to take place in the perceptions of Tanzanian officials about their population problem and appropriate solutions. Of course, this shift did not come out of nowhere. It was embedded in a changed way of thinking about Tanzania's overall approach to development. The formulation of the national population policy involved the intersection of government, donors, and international organizations. Diverse organizations with different but convergent goals gained influence in Tanzania simultaneously, so while this did not have the overt intention of a common front organized to bombard the government with antinatalist propaganda, it did have that outcome. Therefore, we cannot talk about the history of the policy without placing it in the context of the specific relations between the Tanzanian government and its donors and lenders.

Population Policy and Economic Reform

The conflicts over Tanzania's population policy throughout the 1980s are intricately linked with the political and economic constraints on the Tanzanian state as it attempted to negotiate the results of its economic collapse. One informant suggested: "Tanzania was forced into a policy by conditionalities which are not written down because donors want to control population if they are to give aid."[7] This section describes the World Bank's push for population control and then substantiates the relationship between the population policy and economic imperatives. Harrison (2001) describes the politics of adjustment as constituting a framework of the ongoing power wielded by international financial institutions by virtue of states' "permanent crisis" of indebtedness. This web of relationships, both historical and ongoing, is an important component of analysis for policy implementation. The gendered impact of structural adjustment is well-documented in theoretical analyses (Elson 1991, 1995; Palmer 1992) and empirical studies (Afshar and Dennis 1992; Beneria and Feldman 1992; Cagatay, Elson, et al. 1995; Gladwin 1991). However, these disparities are rarely linked with the objectives of population policy. Nonetheless, in Third World development, many of the major proponents of economic liberalization—individual and institutional—are the same as those advocating population policies, and the countries targeted by these policies are identical.

The World Bank is clearly a significant institutional actor in promoting economic liberalization, and while the Bank has become a player in health care reform (see Standing 2002), it is not usually considered to be among the most powerful actors in the population field. Yet, perhaps because the Bank is not associated with promoting a population-control agenda, it is able to push for these goals without incurring the same backlash that might be aimed against stronger population actors. Gibbon's (1991) work suggested that the Bank has long embraced population control as one of its regulatory measures used in the Third World. The Bank laid out a popularized version of its role in population issues in "Population and Development: Implications for the World Bank" (1994).[8] Here the Bank points to the "political acceptability of fertility regulation" as the "most critical issue to address" in poor countries (World Bank 1994, 86). The Bank also notes: "donor influence has to be used judiciously to increase political and public sensitivity to the health and welfare hazards of unrestrained reproduction" (Ibid.).

The World Bank's role in problematizing population has looked similar throughout Africa. Williams' (1995) study of discourses on population, agriculture, and environment demonstrates that "the basic diagnoses and policy recommendations of all these documents are remarkably consistent with the policies and practices which the World Bank has espoused since its foundations" (Ibid., 173). Williams shows how the Bank ignores both historical evidence and geographical variation, instead representing all of Africa "as deriving from a generic process engendered by the reproductive and economic activities of numerous people, activities whose adverse consequences they neither intend nor recognize" (Ibid.). The Bank's representation of Africa as a catastrophe of overpopulation, agricultural crisis, and environmental degradation, and of Africans as neither understanding nor controlling these processes, calls forth the development experts to cope with the crises and promote the common good.

By the mid-1980s, almost no government funds were available for financing the development or implementation of the National Population Policy. The state acknowledges that "due to these budget difficulties the national population programme is mainly financed by multilateral and bilateral assistance" (United Republic of Tanzania 1994, 28). Therefore, the Tanzanian National Population Policy was, from its inception, a policy that would be dependent on donor funding and shaped by donor interests. There are varying interpretations of what the lack of government contribution signifies. It may be an indicator of insufficient political commitment toward the population issue (as it has been understood at various times by donors and analysts in Tanzania), or it may be that the Tanzanian government is simply being strategic by putting its money into areas where donors are less readily available, given that external funds for population issues may be more easily forthcoming (see Richey 1999).

We do know that the history of Tanzania's relationship with international donors and lenders includes population. Tanzania's population issues were taken up in the first Paris Club meetings between the state and international lenders. The World Bank statement given at the Consultative Group for Tanzania meeting in June 1986, the first of such meetings since 1977, stated:

> We also expect to initiate studies on longer term issues such as education and training needs in Tanzania, and we will in response to the minister's request examine the possibility of support in the population field (World Bank 1986, 3, 4).

In the previous quote, the Bank uses careful language to avoid any possible implications that its policies had an impact on the decision of the government to develop a national population policy. Yet, as quoted in the beginning of this discussion, there was a perception in Tanzania that the policy was imposed by the country's donors and lenders.

The World Bank Social Sector representative at the Dar es Salaam Mission Office stated in an interview that he "could not remember" if the Bank had been involved in any way with the formulation of the National Population Policy, but he did not think that they had been involved.[9] He also stated that the Bank was supporting a health and nutrition project worth $47 million, including a "tiny component to support the Population Planning Unit [part of the Planning Ministry responsible for developing and coordinating population policy]." According to the Bank's data, the "tiny component" was $9.5 million (World Bank 1994, 118). My informant from the Bank explained that the PPU was supposed to have been cofinanced by UNFPA, but due to some "mistake of communication," the Bank ended up financing the whole thing. The position of the World Bank and IMF on Tanzania's population problem is rarely discussed in official documents, as the Bank is reluctant to be identified with pushing for a population policy.

The Bretton Woods institutions' interpretation of whether or not Tanzania had a population problem was initially vague, depending on the context of discussion, but by the late 1980s it was clear that population had begun to be perceived as an impediment to economic development. The 1986 Economic Recovery Programme drafted by the Tanzanian government in collaboration with the World Bank and the IMF stated: "Tanzania is a *relatively thinly-populated country.* There is a place and ample space for large private farms...." (United Republic of Tanzania 1985, 30, emphasis added). However, by the June 1988 report, the need for cost sharing was attributed to the problem of over-population:

> Rehabilitation and development of the [social] sector will also be affected by the expansion of the requirements to the sector given the high rate of population growth. With these problems in mind, the Government is now reviewing how beneficiaries can make a more direct contribution to the financing of such services (United Republic of Tanzania 1988, 8).

When justifying the potential for private enterprise in agriculture, the country was "thinly populated," but when discussing government provision of social services, Tanzania became overpopulated. In 1988, the World Bank's report to the Paris Club meeting stated clearly its interest in Tanzania's population problem:

> In addition to these key priorities for economic management, there are longer term development challenges which face Tanzania. *Among these are the preparation of a population policy,* to reduce over time Tanzania's present high rate of population growth, and to take account of its impact on the urban areas and on the provision of social services. The present growth rate of close to 3 1/2 percent per annum imposes an intolerable strain on basic services, on the labour market and on the environment. *It needs to be brought down to a manageable level as rapidly as possible* (World Bank, 1988, 8, emphasis added).

The World Bank's report to the Paris Club the following year blames deteriorating social services on the population problem and reiterates the need for population control. In this report, the Bank asserts: "Tanzania faces a serious population problem" (World Bank 1989, 20). As a solution, they commend the government's development of a population policy with a strong demographic agenda:

> [T]he Government has developed a national population policy with the objectives of reducing fertility rates by 30 percent by the year

> 2000…reducing the proportion of women marrying before the age of 20, minimum spacing of 2 years between births, and attaining a higher contraceptive prevalence. To achieve these objectives and more, over the coming years it will be necessary for Government and for donors to concentrate efforts on expanding family planning services and provision of contraceptives throughout the country…." (World Bank 1989, 21).

The Bank here clearly spells out what it wanted in a population policy, namely, specific targets for lowering fertility. The World Bank's 1989 report to the Paris Club also blames population growth for the government's inability to provide basic social services (World Bank, 1989, 8).

Interestingly, in the period between the 1988 and 1989 reports, the population growth rate supposedly had *decreased* (without the help of a population policy) from 3.5 percent to 2.8 percent, but this was given no explanation. Such a dramatic drop in rates of growth in one year would be impossible. Of course, a likely scenario is simply that a different source of adjusted data was used; however, it would seem that for the Bank, the "real" population growth rate was a question of expediency, not one of correct data. While it might be difficult to prove that Tanzania's structural adjustment loans were held hostage until a population policy was agreed upon by the government, this was the case for Egypt (see Kaplan 1976 cited in Morsy 1995, 165) and Kenya (see Hodgson and Watkins 1997). The Bank's statements as those cited above suggest that there was more than a casual relationship between the World Bank activities in Tanzania and the preparation of a particular kind of population policy to bring down Tanzania's population growth rate.

As the donors and lenders began to point to a population problem, the Tanzanian state responded accordingly. The report prepared by the government addressed the Bank's abrupt concern with population:

> Given the critical role of population-related programmes in overall socio-economic development, the Government has finalized the preparation of a population policy which will be adopted during the ESAP period. The main goals of the national population policy are to reinforce national development…More specifically, the population policy will initially concentrate on expanding and strengthening maternal and child health and family planning programmes (United Republic of Tanzania 1989, 15).

Similarly, the statement given by the Tanzanian finance minister promised, "Population issues will also receive special attention under ERP II" (Ibid. 1989, 10).

However, to the displeasure of its donors and lenders, the government engaged in strategic foot-dragging that prolonged the actual adoption of the policy by over a year. By 1991 when the National Population Policy was still not finalized, the report prepared by the government for the consultative group meeting in Paris in June reassured the lenders that: "In population, the Government has prepared and this year will formally adopt and announce its population policy for the 1990s" (United Republic of Tanzania 1991, 5). When I asked a government official directly involved with the policy why he thought that Tanzania's donors wanted a particular type of national policy so quickly, he responded with two words: "bilateral relationships."[10] He elaborated:

> Donor countries are not merely philanthropic, committed to assisting the poor. Behind that assistance there are things which are of interest to their countries. Population elements are important to them. What happens in other countries will have an impact if not today, then later...It is hard to say why they do things. Many of us have no access to information beyond project documents. We are grateful to donors. We believe it should not be of our concern what is behind it. As long as it doesn't affect us, we make the best of what is given.[11]

Tanzanian State Represents Population Problems in International Fora

The Tanzanian state could not be seen as simply capitulating to donor and lender demands on population issues. In the early 1980s, the Tanzanian government was continuing with its implicit population policy, while subtly but steadfastly refusing to succumb to donors' preferences for an official population policy or family planning. The official stance is demonstrated through the regular reporting mechanism of countries to the Economic Commission for Africa (ECA) Population Division Inquiry on population as shown in table 2.1. Tanzania reported to the ECA in 1977, 1979, and 1981 the state's perceptions that population growth and fertility rates were satisfactory. However, the next year the tone changed.[12] By this time in the economic crisis and the international population consensus, Tanzania could not claim that population was not a problem, but they could give their own prioritization of what kind of problem it was thought

Table 2.1 Summary Information of Tanzanian Responses from UN Monitoring Reports for All Independent African States

Issue	*1977*	*1979*	*1981*	*1983*	*1987*
Population growth	Maintain rates	Maintain rates	Maintain rates	Lower rates desirable, but only some support is appropriate	Lower rates desirable, but only some support is appropriate
Fertility levels	Maintain rates	Maintain rates	Maintain rates	Maintain rates	Maintain rates
Rural-urban flows	Lower rates	Lower rates	Lower rates	Lower rates	Lower rates

Source: Ekanem (1988, 18).

to be. By the 1987 report, the government again reported that fertility rates were too high, but continued to insist that policies to lower it would be inappropriate (United Nations Economic Commission for Africa 1989, 18). This stance was held until the postpolicy reports to ECA in 1996 and 2001 where Tanzania asserted that its population and fertility were "too high" and policies had been put in place to lower them.[13]

Also, in international conferences as in ECA reporting, the genesis of the population policy was linked to government priorities. These international conferences were highly politicized jousts over the meaning and significance of a population problem, and Tanzanian national perspectives both contributed to the international debate and were shaped by it. For example, Tanzania's report to the Third African Population Conference claimed that the ruling party itself was taking on the population concern:

> In the 1980s, Chama Cha Mapinduzi (CCM) and its Governments became more concerned with the implications of population growth for the achievement of various economic goals and national development. Hence, in 1986, programmes to educate CCM and Government leaders on the relationship between the population growth trend and national development were instituted (United Nations Economic Commission for Africa 1992, 64).

In the previous statement, it appears that the party was in charge of defining the problem and asking for education, yet as we will see, these seminars were actually sensitization exercise to help Tanzanians to tow the neo-Malthusian line on its population problem. Still, it was important that the state appear in charge of its own policy agenda.

Sensitizing the Tanzanian State

The 1980s were spent trying to raise awareness about population issues in the country (Overseas Development Administration 1991, 4). These awareness creation seminars, workshops, and national conferences were simultaneously arenas for and actors in shaping the discourse of population in Tanzania. The party, its governments, and NGOs were all involved in consciousness raising seminars. These seminars also served as "another mechanism used to assess the national perceptions of population issues...conducted since in the late 1970s" (United Nations Economic Commission for Africa 1992, 64).

The problematization of population had to be presented to policymakers, government officials who would implement the policies (particularly those in the Ministry of Health since they would be responsible for family planning), and individuals who would ultimately be making the fertility decisions determining population growth. A series of seminars were organized by UMATI with UNFPA and Pathfinder funding, and at the behest of the ruling party Chama Cha Mapinduzi (CCM), beginning in 1984 and running throughout the late 1980s. These seminars were supposed to provide a forum for exchanging ideas, but they were, in fact, focused more on consciousness raising. At these seminars, local experts from the Ministry of Health and the University of Dar es Salaam (UDSM) who were thinking demographically presented papers on the various problems posed by population growth in Tanzania. For example, a seminar on Population and Development was held in Arusha in 1984. According to the Information Sheet for Participants, the "major objective of this seminar is to provide a forum to discuss and exchange ideas on issues related to population family planning and socio-economic development" (UMATI 1984, 2). Even though the seminar title was the same as one held in 1980, its content had changed dramatically. The same words were being used, but their referents had changed. The emphasis on family planning was clear, as was the need to reduce population growth.

In a paper presented by a senior medical officer from the Ministry of Health, the individual level health benefits and the national level issues of health budgets were conflated to produce a win-win scenario (Urrio 1984).[14] He gave the same goals as presented in earlier portrayals of what the Tanzanian government saw as its problem—quality social services, employment, and migration—but instead presented the "new" solution of "lowering population growth." Another paper elaborated that Tanzania "should realize that rapid population growth rates are important constraints to social and economic growth, and that these rapid growth rates largely result from high fertility. Hence, the need to formulate appropriate population policies which aim at reducing fertility and consequently the growth rates" (Sembajwe 1984, i). A new category has been created. The realm of "appropriate" population policies is now clearly defined and quite narrow in its scope. Where previously claims were made that any government policies aimed at impacting either quality or quantity issues were indeed "population policies," now the discourse is more transparent in disclosing that real population policies are designed to bring down fertility.

However, the shift from a development approach to a demographic one was neither immediately nor unilaterally accepted by Tanzanians, and thus more seminars were held. A funding request from UMATI included the following justification:

> Some key policy makers in the country, and especially the President Mwalimu J.K. Nyerere have realised the negative trend at which population and socio-economic trends have been taking and have exhorted the nation to balance reproduction and resource availability [*sic*]. Unfortunately the reaction by the bodies concerned to curb this trend has been minimal. Little has been done to incorporate population variables into the planning system by planners of socio-economic programmes. Even though the Ministry of Health supports family planning, it does so more as a means of maintaining health of the family than for demographic reasons (Nsekela 1985, 1).

The goals of these seminars were no longer phrased in the rhetoric of "sharing perspectives" but were now intended to "help in the establishment of population policy and increased support for UMATI by the policy-makers in the country"(Nsekela 1985). The most critical seminar was conducted in Dar es Salaam in November 1986 for members of CCM, the National Executive Committee, ministers of both the Union and Zanzibar governments and members of the Zanzibar Revolutionary Council. It was chaired by former President Nyerere, and its proceedings instructed the government to come up with a national population policy, stating:

> Tanzania is ripe for a policy on population which will serve as a guideline for general directives and orientations on the relationship between

> the rise in population growth and the rise in the GDP. The aims and objectives of the policy should be to raise the living standards of the people (Goppel 1987).[15]

Also included amongst the 18 recommendations was "Unplanned births have adversely affected socio-economic development, child and mother health and overall family welfare. To solve the above situation, the seminar stresses the need for family planning" (Goppel 1987). The official stance had been signaled clearly with the intention of a population policy that linked population growth, unplanned births, and family planning. This shift did not go unnoticed in the media. A news article reported:

> The ruling Chama Cha Mapinduzi called a three-day seminar to educate Cabinet ministers on the issue. Widespread agreement was expressed at the seminar on the problems involved in catering for 800,000 new mouths a year, and the danger, in the words of a Finance Ministry official, of 'social chaos because resources will be exhausted and pressure on the land increased.' But the battle is not over. A senior economist from the Ministry of Finance and Planning, U.P.K. Tenende, stressed that economic growth could not be attained simply by lowering the population growth rate (Lenga 1987).

Battle lines had been drawn, even though it seemed that all the voices in the government were not speaking at the same volume. Some high-ranking officials were emphasizing the earlier stance on population and development, while others were eagerly blaming the nation's problems on the evils of population growth. The same news article concluded: "Although planners nervously rebut accusations that they want to restrict family size, it is significant that the ruling party, legally supreme to the government, has awoken to the dangers of unplanned population growth. It means that the party's opinion-makers can be used to spread the message about the importance of child-spacing" (Lenga 1987).

Once Tanzanians, or at least high-level officials, were seen as holding appropriate perceptions of their population problem, the issue could be discussed separately from the whole gamut of economic and social policies and programs in ways that had been previously impossible. The official approach to population problems was reported as shifting "from population-responsive strategies in the past development plans to the current situation where population-influencing strategies are worked out through the Government's adoption of the national population policy and the formulation of a national implementation programme" (United Nations Economic Commission for Africa 1992, 64). Furthermore, the political struggles that had been at the heart of changing national perceptions disappeared, and the descriptions of the policy history took on a concurring tone.

For example, UNFPA's history of the national policy, quoted here at length for its carefully constructed discourse of consensus states:

> In the early period of Tanzania's independence, government recognized that high rates of population growth could impact socio-economic development especially the development of social services e.g. education, health and provision of employment. Census taking was given priority and family planning was introduced in public health services programmes as part of maternal and child health care. Nevertheless, there were no systematic programmes aimed at reducing rates of population growth. The situation today has however changed. Conscious effort by the Government, with support by UNFPA and other international agencies, has since the early 1980s considerably raised awareness of population issues in national development throughout the Tanzanian community, and concretely place these issues on the public agenda. The Government after itself learning from the experiences of other countries and carefully weighing the evidence about the country itself, concluded that the quality of life of its citizens would be in danger if nothing is done to plan to bring out a balanced relationship between population size and growth and the use of resources, income growth, income distribution etc. in the country (United Nations Population Fund 1994a, 1, 2).

In this version of how the policy came into existence, the policy was simply a formal recognition of what the government had been doing all along with its implicit population policy and combining that with a proper understanding of the problem of population. In spite of official insistence that UNFPA had not been lobbying for a population policy, documents written after the policy had become a fait accompli tell a different story: "During the Second Tanzania Country Programme [1987–1991], one of the three *unofficial priorities* was the formulation and adoption of the National Population Policy. This priority was achieved when the NPP was officially adopted in January 1992" (United Nations Population Fund 1994c, annex E, emphasis added). The objectives discussed in the 1979 UNFPA Needs Assessment report were completed, and Tanzania was to have an explicit population policy to meet its self-defined development needs and goals.

Officially, population was depoliticized and solutions were rational and administrative.

Drafting the National Population Policy

In 1986, The PPU was created in the Department of Human Resources Planning of the Planning Commission as a focal point on population issues and was "charged with the overall responsibility of fostering the . . . mechanisms needed by the nation in order to address *its identified population problems*" (United Nations Population Fund 1994a, 2, emphasis added).[16] This was the first project of this kind in the country, and in its second phase in 1991, UNFPA notes that "key among these was formulation and adoption of a National Population Policy in 1992" (Ibid.). A news article reported that "like many other African governments, the Administration in Tanzania is under increasing pressure to draw up a policy to control what some experts describe as a 'near explosion' of population" (Lenga 1987). In 1987, CCM directed the government to prepare a National Population Policy, and a National Population Committee was set up with a secretariat in the Ministry of Finance, Economic Affairs and Planning.

The writing of the population policy began with the commissioning of background papers in 1987 for review by a technical organization formed to assist the government in drafting a policy, the National Population Committee. This multisectoral committee[17] developed out of the organization of the Second African Population Conference held in 1984 in Arusha. The committee was described during an interview with a university professor participant as "lots of groups from all sectors;" however, in his opinion, all of them except for him, "were focusing on the bad effects of population growth on development."[18] The committee, guided by international consultants, seminars, and study tours in good population policy countries such as Indonesia, came up with a draft for discussion (see United Republic of Tanzania 1994, 7). The government's draft then underwent technical review and revision by international consultants from UNFPA, ILO, and ECA. In 1989, a completed policy was drafted that included numerical demographic targets.[19]

All of these targets were completely written out of the next draft of the policy. One informant said that he had been told that demographic targets were politically unacceptable.[20] Another informant said during an interview that the draft was sent to the UNFPA in New York where it was changed dramatically. The policy was to be general and all targets were to be removed, and saved as part of the implementation. Tanzania's international advisors, such as UNFPA, were attuned to the political sensitivity of population control in Tanzania, and did not want the policy itself to spark any more controversy than necessary. Ironically, once Tanzanians were sensitized to think demographically, their policy targets were more draconian than would have been acceptable to the international organizations pushing for change.

Negotiating the politics of this policy was time consuming, and the donors accused the Tanzanian state of foot-dragging. However, state officials blamed the extent of such a lengthy process of drafting, revising, and officially declaring the policy on the need to combat religious dissent. In 1989–1991 the Union Government organized high-level seminars for religious leaders on the policy issues;[21] two of these were chaired by former President Nyerere, with then President Mwinyi and all top government leaders in attendance. In 1989, CCM decided to present the policy to religious leaders (bishops/archbishops and sheikhs) based throughout the country at seminars held in Dodoma in 1988 and in Zanzibar in 1989. According to a government official who participated, on the last day before the Dodoma seminar was to begin, the organizers decided not to present the policy. They had been informed that the religious right, particularly the Muslims from Zanzibar, were "intent on tearing it up." The religious leaders did attend the requisite meetings on population; however, an informant gave the example that when the first paper was presented in the potentially volatile Dodoma meeting, someone stood up in the audience and said, "*Tumeitika wito*" meaning that they had only come because they were called, but were not ready to discuss the issues. My informant elaborated: "If it were not for the skills of *Mwalimu* [Nyerere] during certain controversial meetings, they would not have gone on for more than an hour."[22]

In 1990, the second meeting of this type was called to bring together religious leaders, but this time the Catholics refused to attend. The Muslims sent representatives, but would not give any input into the policy. In 1990 after the seminars, the Planning Commission worked on the policy and submitted it officially to the cabinet. The procedure was such that even if the government approved, the policy still had to go to the central committee of CCM for approval as final policy. The technical wing of the CCM Central Committee wanted to give their input as well, so meetings were held with the Planning Commission to revise the policy again. The final format of the policy came from this revision and it was sent again to the government in January of 1992.

Formally Adopting the National Policy

The international donors and Tanzanian government continued to juggle the political appropriateness of adopting the policy. It is likely that policy delays were caused by both internal religious dissent and foot-dragging by members of the government. The Tanzanian state found itself caught in between competing demands from strong international interests in favor of the policy, and important domestic interests against it. In 1991, UNFPA funded another series of seminars "to mobilise mass support for the adoption of the NPP" (United Nations Population Fund 1994c, 35).[23]

The National Population Policy document was published by the Planning Commission in the President's Office in March 1992. It looks nearly identical to such policies in other African countries, and its blueprint-led character obfuscates the highly political process of negotiations between diverse national and international interests. However, an informant noted that, in fact, by June 1992, the PPU expected approval from CCM, but the transition to political multipartyism added another layer of bureaucracy onto the process. In July 1992, acceptance was formally announced by the prime minister. Once it became clear to the Tanzanian state that it would be necessary to declare an official policy to signal its participation in the international community on these issues, the timing and process of the policy itself became critical for maintaining ownership of the policy in the eyes of national stakeholders.[24] Neither the donors nor the state were completely content with the pace of the policymaking process: the donors accused the state of foot-dragging, while the state perceived donor haste as counterproductive. One informant said that the Planning Commission continued to postpone meeting on the policy because politicians did not see it as important. "On the agenda, it [population] has always received a low priority."[25] However, the informant expressed that he believed that the issue had been forced by donors. Responding to criticism by British donors over the slow pace of bringing out the policy, the Planning Commission principal secretary said: "Such a policy has to be flexible enough to adapt itself to these concerns and has also to command consensus. Such a policy needs time to formulate" (Overseas Development Administration 1991b, 7).

Even though the timing of the policy and its implementation were not ideal in supporting the work of international population donors, the official policy document embodied state legitimacy for development activities. UNFPA acknowledged that its long history of working toward, or pushing for, a policy had been successful, and outlined that the next step was to focus on implementation: "[I]n consideration of the substantive background work already done for nearly a decade, and the fertile stage reached already, the focus should now shift toward concentrated efforts that must ensure promotion and support to implementation of Government's own policy provisions and their programmes" (United Nations Population Fund 1994a, 4).

With the declaration of a national policy, the Tanzanian state signed onto the international problematization of population as a problem, and as the previous quote illustrates, it was important for the other participants in the policymaking process to be able to claim that it was nonetheless "the government's own policy." The then minister of state President's Office and vice chairman of the Planning Commission, Horace Kolimba, summed up what the state had agreed to:

> With the adoption of the national population policy Tanzania is committed to solve problems related to rapid population growth, especially initiating measures and programmes aimed at reducing the rate of the country's population growth (United Republic of Tanzania 1994, i).

Such a commitment by the Tanzanian state seems unsurprising in the contemporary context where most African countries have adopted population policies aimed at reducing population growth through fertility control. However, in the context of a different vision of the problem of population as understood by some Tanzanian leaders throughout the policy debates, the policy demonstrates that the goals of changing the perspective of the Tanzanian state on population issues were met. Still, the existence of an explicit national population policy does not mean that the theoretical and ideological debates over defining issues of population have been resolved. Instead, in the words of Knippers-Black, "the ambiguities, inconsistencies, and outright but unacknowledged conflicts are pushed out of the assembly rooms and boardrooms and into the field" (Black 1991, 139). The extent of the discourse shift did not go unnoticed by Tanzanians involved in the policy process itself. A professor from the UDSM explained the meaning of such a shift for his colleagues. He and a prominent government statistician were the first to specialize in demography in the country, and at that time he explained, "people thought we must be stooges of imperialism." Then, to his astonishment, "by 1987, CCM calls and says that they want a National Population Policy within six months!"[26]

What the Policy Says: Competing Discourses in the Text

The official announcement of the National Population Policy signified the triumph of the international organizations and donors in reinterpreting the discourse of population such that the Tanzanian government had recognized its problem. The population literature usually measures explicit political support on the basis of statements made by leaders and by the existence of a national policy. In spite of their blueprint-like generic character, explicit national policies differ from each other in important respects (Heckel 1986). Thus, it is not merely the existence of a policy but the mechanisms for its implementation that must be analyzed to determine the level and character of political support for population issues. Indeed, the actual policy document is a vague and extremely broad statement. Instead of fully embracing the demographic narrative, or clinging to earlier stances on the importance of the development problem, it includes both. The ambivalences and disagreements over the causes and solutions proposed to Tanzania's population problem are represented in the text itself and even more strikingly in its implementation. The following discussion turns to the text of the policy document to understand how it manifests the politics that surrounded its formulation.

The National Population Policy document, 40 pages in length, was published by the Planning Commission in the President's Office in March 1992. The foreword to the document, written by the prime minister and first vice president Hon. J.S. Malecela, begins by emphatically linking the problem of population with larger issues of development: "[t]he main goal of the National Population Policy is to extend the horizon of the country's development plans whose principal objective is to move Tanzanians away from poverty and extend their horizon of standard of living" (United Republic of Tanzania 1992, iii). Malecela goes on to describe Tanzania's 30-year history of dealing with population issues—their implicit population policy. He says that progress made in health care has led to falling mortality rates such that "the population growth rate has been increasing from under 2 percent per year in the 1950's to about 3 percent in the 1980s" (Ibid.). He further notes that "this increase in the population—as explained in this policy—together with the poor technology used by Tanzanians has shown adverse impact on various sectors of the economy and the country's environment" (Ibid., iv). Despite the rhetoric of a government historically and presently concerned only with larger issues of development, the image presented from this statement by the country's second highest ranking political official is one of growing numbers of backward masses with hand hoes, responsible for both economic and environmental difficulties.

The preface to the policy was written by Hon. S.A. Kibona, vice chairman of the Planning Commission and minister of state. He too begins with a link between the policy and development goals of the Arusha Declaration; however, his interpretation is that Tanzanian women need to have fewer children. He gives statistics on the Gross Domestic Product (GDP), concluding that "it is evident that the high population growth rate contributes to the low rate of increase of GDP per capita in the country" (Ibid., v). Of course, the not so subtle implication is that to raise GDP per capita, to increase development, it is necessary to decrease the number of people. This is an example of how in the population discourse, things that are mathematically true, that is, in a proportional relationship, increasing the denominator yields a smaller overall number, are used to imply expanded truths as self-evident when they are actually debatable political questions. Indeed, increasing population does mathematically reduce the GDP per capita; however, the implied relationship, that somehow increasing population is a detriment to development in a larger sense—that increasing population is "bad" and will lead necessarily to poverty—is not well founded. The relationship between numbers of people and levels of economic production is far more complex than simply an arithmetic formula; it involves the existence of opportunity structures that permit the realization of economic potential. As discussed by Hartmann (1995), Furedi (1997), and others, simply decreasing numbers of poor people does not mean that there is less poverty.

The contradictions between demographic goals and development goals of the national policy are seen throughout the policy itself. Because any government that tells its people that they are too many is likely to be met with resistance, Kibona ends with a disclaimer. He says: "The government and the people of the United Republic of Tanzania intend to deal with population growth problems in the best ways possible and which are acceptable to the society. The implementation of this policy therefore will respect individuals' human rights and religious beliefs" (Ibid., vii). This statement provides assurance to powerful dissenters as described earlier.

Throughout the policy, there is an assumption that fertility levels and thus population growth rates are changeable, while other areas of development such as the provision of social services are constant.

"The data from past censuses show that a positive and significant relationship exists between fertility and population growth rate *if infant mortality, urbanization and literacy levels do not change*" (Ibid., 1, emphasis added). Why should we assume that change is not only possible but likely in areas of fertility control, while other areas are projected to remain the same? The unstated assumption is that these issues require major transformations and interventions, but fertility levels are more accessible and amenable to supposedly apolitical inputs such as the provision of family planning services.

The policy section dealing with "Sources of Population Growth" actually deals with only one source: high fertility levels. It points out that "fertility is estimated to have remained constant over the past three decades" and then goes on to cite Tanzania's crude birth rate and total fertility rate in comparison with these rates overall in the world. It is not my point to argue that the fertility level of Tanzanian women is low, or even desirable, but rather to show that a particular scale of analysis, looking at comparisons and cost-benefits from a macro-level perspective of population simply obscures the realities of these issues for people (see Scott 1998). What is "high" fertility in the Tanzanian context? There is no reason why one should assume that fertility rates could or should be standardized around the world, irrespective of issues of culture, consumption patterns, or resource availability. The first two sections of the policy appear to have been written from a point of consensus over the existence of high population growth rates attributable to high fertility rates. However the third section, "Consequences of Rapid Population Growth" is crucial, because it is in this section that the official policy must take a stand on what the results of this population growth are, that is, to what extent is population growth a problem for development. The policy states:

> The national economy did not grow significantly in the last decade because of various constraints, although it has started picking up in recent years. As a result, the resources available per head had declined by between 7.5–10 per cent during 1980–85, and increased by 1.0 per cent per annum between 1985–91. This, of course, does not imply any simple cause and effect relationship between population growth and the national product. Population growth is not the primary obstacle to development but it aggravates the situation and renders remedial measures more difficult (United Republic of Tanzania 1992, 6).

Here we see the policy language shift from statistical truth, to a more qualified and nuanced perception of the relationship between population and development. However, just as we might begin to conclude that the previous quotation represents the "real" position of the Tanzanian government, after an earlier nod to external pressures in the policy, the next paragraph returns specifically to cost-benefit rhetoric and to solving the population problem as a prerequisite for development.

Demographic and development narratives are again given an odd juxtaposition as the discussion then blames underdevelopment on structural adjustment policies. The entire international economic system is now under scrutiny from the population policy:

> 18. On the other hand, macro-economic policies such as those under the structural adjustment programmes have a direct, sharp and immediate impact on the quality of life of the population. Such programmes entail: i. Reduction of public expenditure in the sensitive and basic sectors of health, education and nutrition, etc.; ii. Sudden rises in prices of essential consumer goods; iii. Retrenchment of workers.
>
> 19. The primary concerns of the population policy are: i. To safeguard, as much as possible, the satisfaction of the basic needs of the vulnerable groups in the population; ii. The development of human resources for current and future national socio-economic progress (Ibid., 7, 8).

The above quotations are unusual because they show an abrupt break with preceding discussions of the typical population problem. This language and ideology could have been taken straight out of the 1970s Bucharest discourse. Thus, this dual policy discourse suggests that the government is actually not fence sitting, but more likely, playing both sides or giving a polyvalent performance: promoting both demographic and development approaches to population.

This is also exemplified by the final section of this chapter entitled, "Goals of the National Population Policy." The first two sentences clearly demarcate where the policy is expected to operate:

> This National Population Policy has as its principal objective to reinforce national development through developing available resources, in order to improve the quality of life of the people. Special emphasis shall be laid on regulating population growth rate, enhancing population quality, and improving the health and welfare of women and children (Ibid., 8).

It is interesting that the "quality of life" goal is mentioned as the "principal objective" and then again just after "regulating population growth rate," as if it were necessary to insert buffers around the demographic goal of population reduction. Perhaps this is also a slight nod to the feminist narratives that by this time had become part of the global discourse on population. Until now, women as actors and gender as concept were both conspicuous in their absence from the National Population Policy. However, concluding this section with an emphasis on "improving the health and welfare of women and children" is not as clear cut as it might seem, because while sometimes this terminology is used to refer to larger areas of primary health care, at other times it is simply a euphemism for access to modern contraceptive services.

Chapter two of the policy is meant to outline specifically how population growth will negatively affect the development capacity in particular sectors. In fact, the chapter presents a confused picture of whether population was historically increasing or declining,[27] regional differentiation and population growth attributable to urbanization, not lack of fertility control.[28] My point is not to suggest that the writers of the policy were unable to read and interpret their data correctly, but to show how a particular understanding of the population problem had to be constructed to justify a specific approach taken to deal with that problem. It would have been far more difficult to gain support for the demographic goals of a population policy if the policy clearly stated that between 1978 and 1988, the annual population growth rate dropped, without the aid of any explicit population policy. It would also be a sign of improper recognition of Tanzania's population problem if the document clearly stated that regions experiencing the highest rates of growth are expanding due to migration, not procreation.

Chapter three of the policy deals with "Problems of Special Groups in the Society"—women, children, the youth, the elderly, and the disabled—effectively, everyone except able-bodied, middle aged men. This chapter seems incongruous with the others, as it rarely makes links between the issues it addresses and rapid population growth. In fact, it is a very broad reiteration of development problems, many of which are already covered in policies relating to the specific sectors under consideration. I would argue that this chapter is in the policy as an attempt to assert the breadth of the policy scope—to give specific areas in which the policy is not *just* family planning. It seems out of place within the policy because it is based on a different logic and operates within a different discourse than most of the other sections. The fact that it is included in the final policy document may suggest a refusal to abandon completely the developmental approach of the 1970s.

The final chapter defines the goals of the policy within the appropriate implementing sectors.[29] The recommendations range from very specific—such as "to raise the minimum age at marriage for girls to 18"—to very general—such as "to take measures to mitigate problems of low income and loneliness of the elderly and the disabled." Institutions within the governmental structure that will be responsible for implementation under each section are clearly stated; however, no nongovernmental or intergovernmental organizations are mentioned. The conclusion is brief, but it clearly reiterates the dual discourse of population problematization. It begins with the statement that "An effective implementation of the National Population Policy will mitigate and possibly wipe out socio-economic development problems, caused by rapid increase of the population in the country" (Ibid., 38, 39). However, after confidently stating that population increase has caused the socioeconomic development problems and thus the policy has the potential to solve these, there is again a sort of disclaimer. It states: "The government and the people of Tanzania are committed to solving the problems caused by the rapid population increase, through strategies acceptable to the Tanzanian society, and by paying due attention to and respecting human rights and religious beliefs" (Ibid., 39). So even in the conclusion, we are left with the idea that the discourse on population has changed in such a way that it is now viewed as a problem for development; however, the ways in which this will be handled will still have to be "acceptable to the Tanzanian society" providing an exit option at the stage of implementation if the measures taken are feared to bring forth an unfavorable response.

Conclusions

That the stooges of imperialism from the early 1980s were transformed into national policymakers by the end of the decade speaks to the extent of the official discourse shift in the country. Through discussions with its donors and lenders, sensitization seminars and workshops, and international development missions, the Tanzanian state was convinced to orient its perceptions and policies into line with the global discourse on the population problem. However, while the official discourse has been smoothed against the pumice of international pressure, the conflicting interpretations of causality between population and development have not been eliminated.

A detailed documentation of the politics of this period points to the mediating mechanisms that govern the interactions between abstract centrally promoted plans and social life on the small scale (Tilly 1999)—in this case, between global population discourse and national policy narratives. Throughout the period discussed in this chapter, the Tanzanian state's strategic ambiguity between its own policies and the desires of its donors and lenders has been a polyvalent performance involving "the collective presentation of gestures simultaneously to two or more audiences in ways that code differently within the audiences" (Ibid.). To its constituents, the state was taking a perspective on population that descended directly from its early-independence policies on social service provision in health and education. To its donors, it was taking one showing an understanding of the ways that population growth was impeding national development efforts in just the same areas. To other developing countries, Tanzania was a leader in independent path-making for development, while it was, to varying degrees, towing the line on the global population problem.

However, Tanzania's policymaking relied on an interpretive translation of the global population discourse, and its relationship with donors and lenders is more adequately characterized as accommodative bargaining than as capitulation. Tilly's (1999) redundant phrase is a reminder that bargaining implies give and take on all sides, and includes multiple relations that extend beyond the immediate bargainers exercise of power. The ongoing sensitization seminars, struggles over including or excluding certain objectives or targets, and implicit or explicit support for the interventions of donors or UMATI, all involve a process of accommodative bargaining that is permeated by geopolitical realities. Donors are needed to provide money, UMATI is needed as an experienced implementer, and the government is needed for its legitimacy in policies and institutions. While it may seem that international donors are simply calling the tune for all population interventions, they were constantly forced, often to their displeasure, to accommodate multiple, and sometimes disparate, positions of the Tanzanian state.

There is still not a universal consensus on what a population policy should do in Tanzania and on the role of family planning. These conflicts, ambiguities, and nuances will reappear in the following chapters' discussions of the policy implementation and family planning clinic–level interactions. Government representatives reiterated the importance of clarifying the state's priorities and agenda to counter agenda introduced from other interests—particularly donors. In the words of one high-ranking Tanzanian official:

> It is important to develop strategies that show that [the Tanzanian government] understands all aspects of the population problem. Each country or donor has its own interests in decreasing population growth...We must develop a Tanzanian plan or we will be subjected to universal solutions...reducing the population growth rate is not the central feature of the policy, but at the lower level and the national level, interests may not coincide one hundred percent (Interview 95GD01b, August 13, 1995).

The international politics of donors and recipients in Tanzania's population arena have been analyzed in this chapter. The meaning of population in the discourse as well as the policy itself is vague. This is functional in allowing strategic interpretations that are context-sensitive. In this national context, it is understandable that population may be a more politically palatable concept than family planning. However, family planning is one of the determinants of fertility, which is amenable to large-scale inputs of capital, control from above, and less-partisan political activity; it is, hence, a prime arena for development assistance. This status is unlike that of other significant variables, such as status of women or structure of the economy. This may be the reason why in debates about the population policy in Tanzania, family planning is a more difficult topic on which to gain consensus than population as interpreted as a holistic development issue. However, what is missing in all of these debates is the feminist narrative focusing on gender equality, women's empowerment, choice, and rights. Because of the particular historical context of Tanzania's debates, we still see Malthus versus Marx, the demographic versus the development agenda with little or no reference to local women or to global gender initiatives.

Intermezzo 1

An Interview at the Ministry of Health

Early in my fieldwork, I managed to get an appointment with one of the members of the Family Planning Unit of the Ministry of Health. The unit was then housed in the COSTECH (commission for science and technology) building, a concrete sky-scraper of sorts, sitting behind a muddy parking lot just off the Old Bagamoyo Road between town and the university. The building marked a popular *dala dala* [taxi] stop called *Siansi* [the Kiswahili pronunciation of "science"]. I was deep in the "soaking and poking" phase of my methodology, and so I asked for a lot of clarifications and explanations of things that I would later come to take for granted. Looking back on my fieldnotes from this interview, I think that I may have learned as much from what I did not learn as from the information that I was able to gather. I share the interview in extended form in an attempt to share not only the "back-stage" behavior, but also the scene assembly and prop changes. My informant was extremely well-trained, knowledgeable about international family planning and its Tanzanian variants, and interested in research in general. She had spent a short time on a training visit at my university in the United States, giving her familiarity with my *nyumbani kabisa* [home]. Thus, she was probably willing to spend more time with my incessant and somewhat naïve questioning than other Ministry of Health personnel may have been. She has since left her former position, and thus, my story should not pose any threat of negative professional ramifications; nevertheless, I have changed all distinguishing details to conceal my informant's actual identity.

After exchanging greetings with the slightly surly young woman at the "information desk" at the building entrance, I climbed the cement stairs up to the floor rented by USAID to house the FPU. I noticed the roar of window air conditioners in some offices. Sweating as I climbed, I tried to adjust my jacket and skirt to look professional before calling "*hodi*" and knocking at the door. I was welcomed into the office of my informant, and I took out my list of guiding questions and started interviewing. When I asked about the relationship between the Ministry of Health and the PPU of the Planning Commission, my informant was a bit puzzled. It seemed that she did not really understand "the link" referred to in my question. After a bit of thought, she tried to explain what the link might be. "Formally," she said, "the relationship is between the President's Office and the Ministry of Health, but some projects are multi-sectoral and work in different ministries." She went on to explain that the donors determine the location of a project—"if they are uncomfortable with a person, they will send it to another ministry." I remembered a brief conversation with a USAID consultant whom I bumped into in an office months before while in the United States. He described the head of the PPU as an "obstacle" that had to be overcome in order to promote the population policy in Tanzania. His description was that the Tanzanian official kept stalling projects and did not want to cooperate with USAID's agenda. Now, I can understand a bit more about why the large USAID project sat not in the Planning Commission, but in the Ministry of Health. UNFPA, however, still ran its project through the PPU. Maybe they did not have the same conflict with its head.

During my interview with the Ministry of Health informant, she began an unprompted discussion of the family planning climate change in Tanzania.

> The 1990s changed so much...before you couldn't even talk of family planning, but now there are many changes, liberalization, the international scene—the fall of the Soviet Union. In 1978, UNFPA started consciousness raising, but it had opposition from the church, the feminist movement...then we had a shift from economics to population in terms of development. In Bucharest it never came to the attention of governments that population was an issue...then in Mexico, the US didn't think it was a problem. Now the US government has shifted, and they are trying to push all over the world.

It was interesting to me that the changing climate in Tanzania was explained by a Ministry of Health representative as resulting from geopolitical struggles and shifts—from the collapse of the wall to the rift between American fundamentalists and U.S. delegations to international population conferences. What was left out, of course, was the opinion of Tanzanian governmental delegations, national policy planners, the church, women's organizations, and most of all the Tanzanian women and men who were supposed to be using the newly popular family planning.

However, my informant did bring up the "Tanzanian" side of things when talking about what was important for success in family planning. "Where programs have been successful, you see that the head of state is very involved. That has not been the priority for the head of state here. Probably because he doesn't understand about population as a problem. Some people say it is because he is a Muslim and they are polygamous." Perhaps she noted a quizzical or even disapproving look on my face, because she added: "that's the level people go to when talking about it... but even if they don't get involved, they allow us to do our activities and to promote our programs." In an interesting shift of voice, my informant claimed the activities and programs as "ours."

She went on to explain this notion of what these programs should be:

> We need to combine efforts to promote family planning and poverty alleviation—especially the status of women. To empower women to make the choices available to them—power relations between the sexes is a serious problem... "reproductive health" is a serious problem.

I probed for more clarity summarizing that she seemed to be saying that family planning must be linked with development more broadly, and while this happens in theory, what about what happens in practice? "USAID won't even listen to that!" she laughed, "The bulk of USAID funds go to Technical Assistance—they must pay for US consultants." I asked about negotiations between the government and donors, and she said it is not like negotiations because donors have all the power. They dictate what will be spent and where. She discussed the dilemma of donor priorities that differ from others:

> Can you improve the quality of family planning without improving the rest of the services in health care? Can you really expect to give everything to one child in the family and help the whole family? If AVSC[1] gives these machines to a clinic, but they can only be used for one thing, and a mother comes in with complications from a pregnancy, etc., how can you manage with that? Supplies come from donors for particular uses only, and these high tech supplies are brought into poor hospitals that are running out of everything.

Our conversation was interrupted by two representatives from Macro International, the company that ran the DHS. They introduced themselves jokingly to me as "Beltway Bandits" who were trying to sort out an upcoming meeting for preparing the next DHS questionnaire. They lamented a surplus in their budget that they could not find any way to spend. After they left her office, my informant joked about them, and mentioned how typical it is that consultants fly in for a few days and have so much money to spend, but they cannot spend it on things like buying contraceptives.

We discussed the logistics of my research project and she suggested that I would need a formal letter of introduction to work in the Ministry of Health facilities (any public health clinic). Then she said that when I got to each region, I should contact the Regional Medical Officer or the Regional Research Coordinator who would help me with introductions, but would expect between 5,000–10,000 shillings of *chai* [tea] for the day. Can this be right—the highest ranking medical officer in the region will need payment for helping introduce a researcher while the beltway bandits cannot find any way to spend their money? My informant and I shared some laughter and a lot of head nodding, and then she went back to work on the computer on her desk, both of which were marked in stenciled letters "USAID."

3

Population Policy Implementation and Family Planning

Introduction

There is a difference between counting people and counting stones (U.P.K. Tenende, project coordinator of the PPU).

Despite a lack of consensus amongst the Tanzanian government over the role of family planning in the National Population Policy, in implementation it is primarily a policy for family planning. Implementation of the policy, as discussed in chapter two, depends on the funding of donor projects. These projects are part of a global demographic discourse that promotes family planning as the "solution" to "development" problems. These "problems" are created on the basis of "needs" (see Illich 1993) defined by the organizations whose projects are responsible for meeting them. The National Population Policy is unusual in that its major implementing arm, the National Family Planning Programme was developed in 1989, and actually preceded the population policy itself (adopted in 1992). Therefore, when analyzing policy implementation, it is necessary to understand the history of family planning, even as it predates the policy history. While the existence of the national policy has been critical for donors in family planning, there is a need to portray family planning projects as mere technical, and thus apolitical, interventions. Thus, the population issue is ever present, but often left unmentioned in implementation of the family planning and reproductive health.

The scope of the family planning apparatus in Tanzania has changed significantly between the time of the inception of the National

Family Planning Programme and current interventions to promote the expanded agenda of reproductive health. However, the character of these interventions and the mediating mechanisms between global discourse and local women remain consistent. In fact, some of the problems encountered with integrating the non-family planning aspects of the reproductive health agenda are traceable to the ambivalent roots of the program and policy environment. Therefore, it is critical to understand the historical meaning of the family planning context to begin to grasp the contemporary difficulties in Tanzanian reproductive health care.

To examine what family planning looks like a policy outcome, this chapter analyzes the transition from the population problem to that of the family planning solution. The National Population Policy gave a green light to international family planning interventions, but political support was not unambiguous. The next section traces the ongoing conflicts over the extent of the government's commitment to implementing its policy. Then, a history of family planning services in the country, beginning with the establishment of the Family Planning Association of Dar es Salaam in 1959 follows. The discussion examines how the Tanzanian government became more explicitly involved in childspacing as a result of increased assistance from foreign donors. The culmination of this shift resulted in the National Family Planning Programme, the embodiment of the global population discourse in the Tanzanian context. Next, the different organizational actors and interests involved in the program are surveyed. Because family planning is in large part an amalgamation of various donor interests, this discussion describes each donor's role and examines coordination under the program. The next section examines the oldest family planning provider in the country, UMATI, whose role in the constellation of organizations has changed dramatically. The penultimate section describes the success experienced by the National Family Planning Programme and the limitations of the expanded focus on reproductive health.

Groping Carefully or Foot-Dragging?: The Government, Donors, and Implementation

After having approved the National Population Policy, there were still questions about whether the government was actually going to thwart its implementation. One example is that the government appeared reluctant to grant sufficient office space to its PPU. At various review meetings, donors urged the Tanzanian government to provide a conducive working environment for the PPU.[1] The USAID representative blamed the lack of space for the unit's overall inefficiency saying, "Why is PPU not given enough space by the Planning Commission? Give them the facilities, then question them about why they did not coordinate." Tanzania's donors recognized the lack of implementation success, noting for example, "*the question is whether in-depth, extensive Government commitment exists. If it does, why does there seem to be lack of energetic, dynamic leadership to give direction and guidance to the population and development programme effort? Is the problem at the central level or endemic*" (emphasis in original) (United Nations Population Fund 1994c, annex E)? UNFPA goes on to suggest that, if the problem is simply at the top, regional or district population planning units could be established to implement the programs. Unequal levels of involvement between NGOs and donors vis-à-vis the government in implementing various aspects of the policy is an indication of the government's priorities. One informant suggested to me that: "one thing that can assist you in understanding the position of the government is to look at the government budget—how much money are they putting into family planning—none![2] The moment that USAID and UNFPA withdraw, there is no money which will support family planning. They will say, 'we have other priorities.' "[3]

Indeed the issue of which projects under the national policy get funded and by whom is central to understanding the priorities of the policy. Rhetoric and public support for family planning, or for larger development issues, are important, but the bottom line is always a competition for resources. According to UNFPA, "since 1990 more and more population projects have been included in annual plans . . . this is mainly due to the fact that the government is committing more and more resources towards population projects, and because of this Government commitment it is a requirement that projects must be included in annual plans and budget books" (United Nations Population Fund 1994a, 44). However, as late as the end of 1996, the implementation work plans for the policy were still not finalized, and donor documents suggest impatience with the pace (see United Nations Population Fund 1994c, annex E). Technically, this was because of ongoing debates over whether or not they would be included in the rolling plan, which would make implementation obligatory. A professor from the UDSM explained: "Even the position of the government, although it supports family planning, when it comes to implementation, they don't actually support it financially. They don't do the things they promised…rhetoric in politics and what happens in practice are not the same."[4]

Why would the government have agreed to adopt the policy yet refuse to support the sections of government responsible for implementing it? Perhaps, it was a problem of an ineffective bureaucracy that simply could not get requests in the proper form to enable donors to fund aspects of implementation. Or perhaps it is an example of what Scott (1985) has termed "weapons of the weak" at the highest levels. If the Tanzanian government did not want to be seen as completely complicit in implementing a potentially controversial policy, refusing to allow a strong governmental component to be involved helps to relieve the state of the more visible culpability. At the same time, approving the policy and permitting various donors to implement projects of all varieties under its auspices gives the government the opportunity to take credit for any inputs that are perceived as beneficial.

While government officials may have been ambivalent about the role of family planning in the implementation of the policy, donors were not. For example, USAID clearly spelled out: "*The main intention of the NPP is to strengthen FP services, promote the health and welfare of families, and eventually reduce population growth. The major target* of the policy is to reduce the total fertility rate (TFR) from 6.3 (as measured in the 1991 TDHS) to three by the year 2000" (USAID 1994, 7, bold in the original). The main document reflecting the interpretation of the IMF and World Bank around Tanzania's structural adjustment programs of the 1990s states: "This policy aims to assure that population variables are given more consideration in development policy and to reduce birth rates and population growth over the medium term through voluntary regulation of fertility" (United Republic of Tanzania 1991, 38).

According to one donor, well after the policy had been declared some parliamentarians still held "misconceptions, misguidance, even ignorance based on unfounded arguments like you need more children to prosper economically," but he added "these don't hold water now."[5] To insure that all sectors of the government were thinking demographically to create an "enabling environment" for family planning, USAID funded the Resources for the Awareness of Population Impacts on Development (RAPID) project, an interactive computer simulation model presentation.[6] A government informant pointed out that the model's overgeneralized approach did not go unnoticed when the tool was used with his colleagues. He described: "We held a workshop on the RAPID model and invited some professors from the University of Dar es Salaam... when I presented my part of that model,... [a professor] told me,... 'you are divided into two parts—yourself and that part that is involved in the technical gadgets! *Are you sure that you know the complexities and assumptions behind those models?*' And to me, those are appropriate concerns."[7] The RAPID model itself is an instrument of the family planning apparatus that simultaneously acts as a conduit for global population knowledge and creates an identity for those persons wielding the technology. Thus, the model can be considered an identity artifact reproducing power relations in the local context of the National Population Policy. Other technologies function as identity artifacts in the local context of the family planning clinics as chapter five will elaborate. My policy informant considered the implications of the conflict between the assumptions of the RAPID model and those of his colleagues, musing, "Someone said that you should not stand still—you should be moving—but Africa is groping in the dark, and we must grope carefully" (Ibid.).

From the Population Problem to the Family Planning Solution

> *Nimezaa Kwa Mpango Ninalea kwa Maringo [I have planned my births so I am raising my children gracefully] (Slogan on the kangas[8] of the Tanzanian National Family Planning Programme).*

The demographic, development, and feminist lenses for viewing population are often confused and combined within the population discourse. These definitions of population must be considered side by side, used interchangeably, and often conflated altogether for the logic of the population discourse to continue. This is achieved through the use of an argument known to logicians as a fallacy of equivocation. This fallacy takes the following form: 1) all banks have money; 2) every river has two banks; therefore, 3) all rivers have money. The fallacy, of course, is accomplished by changing the meaning of one of the terms of the syllogism in the middle of the implication.[9] In the population discourse, the follow logic appears: 1) maternal mortality/child health/female education/women's status [or any other "quality" issue] are population problems; 2) population problems ["quantity issue"] are solved by increasing family planning; therefore, 3) maternal mortality/child health/female education/women's status/and so on are solved by increasing family planning. In the population fallacy of equivocation, the meaning of "population problems" changes in the middle of the implication but the logic continues to sound reasonable.

When the Tanzanian government states that it is committed to improving women's and children's health, it is admitting that it has a population problem of the demographic sort defined by the population establishment only if this logical bait and switch is used. Statements made by the government along the lines of stressing the importance of preventive health care are used to make claims that the government supports large-scale family planning programs based on the imperatives of population control. For example, the Ministry of Health claimed: "Although Tanzania does not as yet have an explicit population policy, the Party and Government have always shown interest and awareness over the importance of the population issues in development in general and on the health of mothers and young children in particular" (United Republic of Tanzania, Ministry of Health and Social Welfare 1989, 5). Conversely, if the government shows a lack of enthusiasm for these sorts of family planning initiatives, it is criticized for ignoring issues of preventive health. For example, donor correspondence notes Tanzania's weak population policy environment as a potential hurdle for approval of a large USAID family planning project. The donor headquarters warns the Tanzania USAID mission to:

> Take precaution that policy issues related to preventive health and family planning are not ignored during the design phase of the project. Since the government of Tanzania (GOT) has not to date approved a national population policy, ECPR expressed concern that the GOT will avoid over the short run addressing major policy issues affecting delivery of family planning in Tanzania (USAID 1990, annex A, PID Approval Message, 1).

The implication here is that because the government had not yet approved a national population policy, it was ignoring issues of preventive health and family planning.

While government representatives continued to remind me that the National Population Policy was "more than just family planning," Tanzania's donors read the policy as a symbolic gesture to the international community that the government understood its population problem. The existence of a population policy was interpreted by donors, NGOs, and parts of the Ministry of Health as a gesture of political support for family planning. Even without unanimous support for family planning, simply declaring a population policy had the effect of supporting family planning. As shown by Barrett and Tsui, population policies indicate countries' receptivity to outside assistance, flashing the green light to donor agencies seeking appropriate beneficiaries (1999). Their quantitative cross-national study found[10] that the existence of a population policy holds symbolic value for international aid money (Ibid.). The existence of a population policy proved to be the most reliable predictor in both whether a country receives population aid from USAID and how much money it will receive, even figured on a per capita basis. If a country adopts a population policy, it is 12.5 percent more likely to receive USAID funds, and of those countries having received funding, adopting a policy increases the countries' expected assistance nearly threefold (Ibid., 36). In the Tanzanian case, USAID population money increased one and a half times in the year following the official adoption of the National Population Policy and has continued to increase substantially.[11] The ambiguous meaning of the policy as a green light for family planning but at the same time, as more than just family planning comes out of conflicting agendas held by the Tanzanian government and the donors, lenders, and international organizations involved with the policy.[12]

From the 1959 Birth of UMATI to the 1974 Government Involvement in Childspacing

Tanzania was one of the first countries in Africa to initiate family planning activities. In 1959, the organization that would become the Family Planning Association of Tanzania (UMATI) (now *Uzazi na Malezi Bora Tanzania*) began offering services in Dar es Salaam. At that time their clientele was restricted mostly to whites and a few government officials. UMATI was founded as *Chama cha Kupanga Uzazi cha Dar es Salaam* [literally, the family planning association of Dar es Salaam] with a mission to give information about childspacing to the population of Dar es Salaam. While a national family planning association was not formed until 1966, UMATI gradually expanded the range of its activities, but it did so without formal government participation (Thomas 1979, 8). Despite pronatalist rhetoric by the government, it allowed UMATI to operate as an independent organization to provide services for childspacing, justified on maternal and child health grounds. In 1967, UMATI became a national organization, and services were expanded to Mwanza, Arusha, Moshi, and Liuli towns. Two years later, UMATI became a full member of the IPPF.

The controversy surrounding family planning grew as services expanded. Omari describes how UMATI came under fire in the early 1970's from leftists who objected that "modern family planning practices and methods, especially as perpetuated by the multinational corporations, are an imperialist and capitalist tendency and agents which are not supposed to be allowed in a country that is trying to develop a socialist ideology" (Omari 1989, 35). One incident cited was the regional commissioner's closing of all clinics offering modern family planning within Tanga Region. Also, in 1971, the local government closed the UMATI clinic in Babati (Arusha Region) after claiming that population was not a problem.[13]

In 1972, the organization's name was changed to *Chama cha Uzazi na Malezi Bora cha Tanzania* [literally, the family planning and good childrearing association of Tanzania] signifying its expanded focus on childrearing as well as childspacing (Oosterhuis 1989, 7). The name change may have been an attempt to legitimize the organization at a time when it was becoming increasingly controversial. In 1973, UMATI was embroiled in conflict over its continued use of Depo-Provera, a long-lasting contraceptive injection, after this drug had been banned in the United States. One informant, who had been part of the Ministry of Health and later joined UMATI, explained that "people were trying to get used to the pill [oral contraceptives] and then Depo was brought in." He went on to explain how "there are always rumors and controversies" surrounding new methods, but in this case "the problem was that the USFDA [United States Food and Drug Administration] was not approving it, but was pushing it in other countries." In Tanzania, there was "a little USAID assistance through UMATI" followed in the country by negative press. This made UMATI unpopular again, "especially among the politicians." In response, UMATI came out with guidelines on the use of Depo—that it would be administered only by gynecologists, not by regular nurses.[14] The drug was temporarily withdrawn by the government, then reintroduced with restrictions on its usage. My informant concluded that UMATI "convinced the government not to ban it [Depo-Provera] completely. This was a breakthrough—to know that the government trusted UMATI."[15]

Another early controversy came from UMATI's publication of a pamphlet on sex education, which was deemed inappropriate because it dealt with the discussion between adults and children on issues of sexuality. The pamphlet was later banned (United Nations Population Fund 1979, 73). During this time, family planning was under attack in the national press, and this led to intervention from the government. The ruling political party's executive committee declared its support for UMATI and directed the Ministry of Health to assist them in the promotion and delivery of childspacing services. As Omari described it, the issue of family planning divided members of the ruling party, who "ruled against UMATI but directed that ways be found to integrate family planning services into the health delivery system of the country" (Omari 1989, 35).

In 1974, with support from USAID, the government launched an integrated Maternal and Child Health (MCH) Programme which included childspacing activities "because of their perceived beneficial impact on maternal and child health" (United Republic of Tanzania, Ministry of Health and Social Welfare 1989, 3). Childspacing services were to be offered in all MCH facilities in the country. UMATI's role was reduced to providing IEC to the general public, training service providers, and procuring contraceptives and supplies (United Republic of Tanzania 1994, 9). The Tanga clinics were reopened after the Ministry of Health took over family planning service provision in 1974. Throughout the country during the 1970s a popular "political and ideological stand" was that since land is plentiful and labor is needed, there is no need for fertility control. (Omari 1989, 163). Modern family planning was identified with capitalism and imperialism. However, after modern family planning was taken over by the Tanzanian state and integrated into existing MCH clinics, this stance subsided (Omari 1989, 163). Government involvement gave legitimacy to family planning in Tanzania.

Childspacing Services as Part of the National Health Policy

The 1974 introduction of MCH/FP services by the government was part of a National Health Policy, which had evolved in the early 1970s. The policy was based on the 1967 Arusha Declaration's goals of "Socialism and Self Reliance" and reaffirmed by Tanzania's signature on the Alma Ata Declaration. The National Health Policy emphasized rural health development through a focus on conveniently accessible and free preventive care.[16] Hospital expansion was curtailed in favor of meeting the needs of rural health infrastructure. Between 1972 and

1980, the number of health centers rose from about 100 to 239 and the number of dispensaries rose from about 1,500 to 2,600—locating a health unit within walking distance (5 kilometers) of 72 percent of the population (United Republic of Tanzania, Ministry of Health and Social Welfare 1989, 7). Tanzania's National Health Policy fit easily into the primary health care approach advocated for Third World countries at the Alma Ata Conference in 1978. The primary health care approach consisted of a focus on the preventive management of illness, infection and nutritional deficiency, and a reliance on auxiliary health workers and community participation (Kabeer 1994, 189). Childspacing services were included as part of an array of Maternal and Child Health services including immunizations and TB/Leprosy programs.

In 1982, the Ministry of Health conducted an evaluation of childspacing activities and found that only 37 percent of MCH clinics (715 out of 1943 clinics surveyed) were providing childspacing services (United Republic of Tanzania, Ministry of Health and Social Welfare 1989, 3). The evaluation found that contraceptive use was low and that quality of services was weak due to weak managerial skills, inadequate numbers of service personnel trained in family planning techniques, and weak logistical support (United Nations Population Fund 1979, 23). In response, the government launched the National Childspacing Programme in 1985 with funding from UNFPA (United Republic of Tanzania, Ministry of Health and Social Welfare 1989, 3). The program objectives were to improve the health of mothers and children and to raise contraceptive prevalence from 5 percent to 10 percent (United Republic of Tanzania, Ministry of Health and Social Welfare 1989, 4). One Ministry of Health informant said that these projects in the mid-1980s meant that "the program was taking shape, and then it was easier to talk about a population policy. Before that, advocacy was done by UMATI, focusing on politicians concerning issues of population and development, but without having a groundwork of projects it was difficult to get a policy."[17]

Interestingly, while a government informant saw the second half of the 1980s as a time when family planning was building momentum, UNFPA saw it differently:

In early 1988, on the mainland one still referred to "'birthspacing'...For several years UNFPA had sent international consultants to Tanzania to assist the Government to develop a national birthspacing plan; in early 1988 no such plan had been adopted." In fact the second of three unofficial priorities of the Second Country Programme was to assist the Government to adopt a national birthspacing programme. Furthermore, important and influential elements in the Government and academia[18] seemed to have a mixed perspective on 'population' "—some persons thought that Tanzania needed a larger population and that a lower growth rate might be detrimental to the national development effort" (United Nations Population Fund 1994c, annex E).

From the standpoint of the international family planning agenda, things were mostly at a standstill until 1988. Then, a new national project director was appointed who turned everything around. She managed to bring about a National Family Planning Programme with a plan of operations for about $28 million. The government itself also submitted a proposal to UNFPA for a $6.5 million project—the largest project ever submitted for review by the Africa Division, much to the delight of UNFPA.[19] The government perceived its strengths in: "high awareness among Politicians and Senior Government leaders about the benefits of childspacing on the health of mothers and children," the existence of a well-developed health infrastructure and the moral and material support from the government even "in the absence of explicit population policy" (United Republic of Tanzania, Ministry of Health and Social Welfare 1989, 10).

However, while the Ministry of Health saw Tanzanian government support as a "strength" of the existing childspacing program, USAID saw it as deficient. In fact, USAID claimed that one of the "critical constraints to family planning service utilization" still came from the government, noting: "Ambivalence about the merits of FP [family planning] in some GOT [government] quarters in Tanzania, and a distrust of certain contraceptive methods, have delayed the promulgation of a population policy and prompted the adoption of certain restrictive service delivery policies" (USAID 1990, 7). It would seem that USAID and the Tanzanian government did not hold the same expectations about what political support should constitute. The government may have been supporting what it considered to be "family planning," while USAID was expecting support for a different notion.

Yet, the Tanzanian government did recognize problems with its early family planning program including: 1) a clinic based approach that caters mostly to mothers and children and thus excludes single or childless women and men; 2) pill-dominated program because of restrictions on use of Depo Provera (which must be prescribed by a gynecologist) and lack of supplies for other methods; and 3) inadequate logistic support because of lack of transport, poor information systems, and poor supervision (United Republic of Tanzania, Ministry of Health and Social Welfare 1989, 11). However, most of these were attributed to larger economic decline and a deteriorating health care environment. In contrast, USAID emphasized policy measures that needed reform in the national program:

Namely, contraceptives were not permitted for unmarried persons or childless couples; family life education was not introduced in the schools; Depo-Provera could only be prescribed by a gynecologist; and a woman had to have at least three children before an IUD could be inserted. With the launching of the National FP Program in March 1989, these restrictions were lifted and there remain no major policy impediments. However, it will take some time before service providers and the population at large are fully informed of these changes (USAID 1990, 7).

Tanzania's donors were concerned with issues of access to contraceptives, while the government pointed out the inadequacies of overall health care structure.

It is difficult to document how much family planning was actually going on in Tanzania before the National Family Planning Programme took over.[20] Donors were funding projects with family planning components, such as the Integrated Project in Kilimanjaro sponsored by the Japanese Family Planning Organization (JOICFP) and a Community Based-Distribution (CBD) project in Bagamoyo District called the Family Health Project and sponsored by the German Technical Assistance Agency (GTZ). While we can not be certain of the statistics, what seems likely is that before the national program, some childspacing services were being offered in at least two or three of the MCH clinics. However, many contraceptive methods were restricted, service providers were largely untrained, and women were, by and large, not beginning or not continuing to use contraceptives.

Bringing About the National Family Planning Programme

The National Family Planning Programme officially began in 1989 when "the government took all the responsibilities of providing IEC, training of service providers and procurement of contraceptives and supplies" (United Republic of Tanzania 1994, 10). The program refers to all family planning and related activities taking place within the country with the Family Planning Unit as the coordinator (Family Planning Unit 1992, 1). The government attempted to link this program to its goals of improved primary health and economic development to avoid associations with population control or fertility targets. Its plan of operations states:

> Most of the deaths in mothers and children are preventable through improved MCH services and also through improved socio-economic status of women. It is against this background of high but preventable maternal, perinatal and early childhood mortality and morbidity that Government's efforts to promote family planning must be seen. The Ministry of Health and Social Welfare regards family planning as an important and effective intervention for protecting the family and promoting good health of mothers and children (United Republic of Tanzania, Ministry of Health and Social Welfare 1989, 10).

The recognition that improved socioeconomic status of women is an important factor in preventing maternal and child deaths is significant. In this statement the government was situating family planning as a health intervention, not a demographic one. This kind of stance is key to the national interpretation of the feminist narrative that will become central after the Cairo conference in the mid-1990s. However, "women" in this discourse are taken as children's mothers and not as individual holders of reproductive rights or decision-making authority.

The National Family Planning Programme was developed to meet the "overall goal" of "promotion and protection of the health and nutritional status of the family, especially the mothers and children" and to do this, the "broad objective" was "to raise contraceptive acceptance rate from about 7% to 25% by 1993" (United Republic of Tanzania, Ministry of Health and Social Welfare 1989, 14). One of the other objectives was improving the health of mothers and children. It was elaborated as "(a) Reduce the proportion of women having children before the age of 20 years by 20% by 1993 through IEC; (b) introduce Family Life Education (FLE) to 50% of schools and colleges by 1993; (c) increase the proportion of breast-feeding mothers one year post-partum by 20% come 1993; and (d) increase the proportion of couples spacing pregnancies at 3 year intervals by 30%" (United Republic of Tanzania, Ministry of Health and Social Welfare 1989, 14). As with the National Population Policy text discussed in chapter three, this document includes very different foci for family planning with the most prominent objective fitting donor perceptions and the others coming from a perspective on education and primary health care.

"The NFPP Plan of Operations" projected the modern contraceptive prevalence rates shown in table 3.1.

Table 3.1 Government Projections for Contraception

Year	*1989*	*1990*	*1991*	*1992*	*1993*
Contraceptive Prevalence Rate (CPR) (%)	10	15	20	22	25
Number of acceptors	474,720	734,866	1 million	1.2 million	1.3 million

Source: United Republic of Tanzania, Ministry of Health and Social Welfare, 1989.

It is unclear whether these inflated projections reflected the genuine enthusiasm of the Ministry of Health officials at the national level for whom family planning represented a new source of resources and who would not have to actually deal with the messy task of local implementation, or if it is simply a statement for the potential funders. The review of the National Family Planning Programme notes:

> These objectives were over ambitious and most of them...have not been achieved by wide margins....this was literally the first really serious local attempt by the MOH to prepare a long term family planning programme, without much reliable back-up data to assist objective planning; and without the necessary experiences in planning programme management (Mpangile 1994, 15).

An example of how unrealistic these predictions were is that the modern contraceptive prevalence rate in 1994 was still only 11.3 percent (Weinstein et al. 1995, 33). However, as the earlier discussion pointed out, the importance of the Plan of Operations was not so much in its substance, as in its symbolic meaning, as a show of enthusiasm to donors indicating that the Tanzanian government was ready to embrace family planning.

Despite the official launch in 1989, the National Family Planning Programme did not become fully operational until 1991. The reasons for this delay involve the negotiations between the major donors, UNFPA and USAID, and the Tanzanian Government.[21] In sum, responsibilities were shifted away from UMATI and to the MOH, with USAID calling most of the shots.[22] The extent to which the government assumed or denied ownership of family planning activities varied. Informants used the term "NGO" to refer to any organization implementing projects that was not the government. For example, a UNFPA National Programme officer referred to "smaller donors like the British ODA acting like NGOs" when they were implementing projects such as the Mbeya Health project.[23] From these examples, we can see that the donors often become confused with their projects, and the implementing agencies are mistakenly labeled as the ones giving the funds. The confusion on the ground over policy implementation results from the striking similarity between projects, both in terms of philosophy and goals, and in terms of the local contacts hired to run them. Many of these projects have the same funding sources, and thus, exist according to the strategic objectives of a handful of important donors. In this situation, it is difficult to find local discourses as distinct from the global population discourse promoted by international donors.

The key Tanzania-based agencies participating at the inception of the national program were primarily divisions of the Ministry of Health or other government ministries, CCM, Tanzanian trade and professional organizations, church-affiliated organizations, or UMATI.[24] It was symbolically important that the party formally situate itself in support of the National Family Planning Programme to quell doubts about the reticence of political figures to be associated with family planning. Apart from UMATI, these locally based organizations had a limited role in the formulation or implementation of family planning or population policy. Some of these organizations, such as those affiliated with the churches, were simply including family planning services and education as part of the repertoire of services available at their health clinics. It is interesting that CCM was included among participating agencies on the basis of its role in formulating the National Population Policy.

Family Planning Donors and Coordination

> The political acceptability of fertility regulation in these countries [in the early stage of demographic transition] is often difficult but also the most critical issue to address. Donor influence has to be used judiciously to increase political and public sensitivity to the health and welfare hazards of unrestrained reproduction (World Bank 1994, 86, 87).

Family planning in Tanzania has largely been the purview of international family planning organizations.[25] This is due, in part, to a lack of local expertise in the areas needed for intervention, as also because donors tend to fund organizations based in their own countries as part of the donor patronage system. These organizations are all involved with implementation, education, and service provision but some are also donors themselves, allocating money for support of particular projects. Also, while these organizations are all NGOs, as in not being a part of any government, some receive their funding almost exclusively from a governmental organization, USAID.

Because the family planning since its inception has been funded almost exclusively by donor money, to understand Tanzanian local interventions, we must examine donor priorities. Donors funded the National Family Planning Programme in three ways: 1) funding directly to the Family Planning Unit of the Ministry of Health (FPU/MOH); 2) funding that is used by donors directly for purchase of contraceptives, vehicles, and so on; and 3) funding that is channeled directly to technical assistance institutions. Some donors have funded family planning components of larger development interventions or have implemented pilot projects at the district or regional level.[26] The two biggest family planning donors in Tanzania have been UNFPA and USAID. UNFPA began providing population assistance to Tanzania in 1971 through support for publishing census results, teaching obstetrics/gynecology, studies in MCH and childspacing, and a program for better family living and in 1980, the first comprehensive country program was approved.

In a multicountry study of population, the assessment was made: "If one had to pick the donor agency with the strongest total impact on population programs in the developing countries, the choice would be USAID. Not only was AID a vigorous promoter in its own right, it also bought in and used numerous intermediaries" (Warwick 1982, 45). USAID began assistance to the Tanzania social sector in the early 1970s with a MCHA training project, and "following the revitalization of USAID's development program in 1987, a number of discrete activities in support of population and family planning efforts have been initiated." (USAID 1990, 9).

USAID interventions in Tanzania are not unlike its concerns with overpopulation in other parts of the Third World: "Since its inception, the population program within USAID had been devoted primarily, if not exclusively, to demographic goals" (Moffett 1994, 286–287 cited in Hodgson and Watkins 1997). In Tanzania, "successful recovery is dependent upon the productivity of the Tanzanian people; productivity will be severely eroded by the consequences of uncontrolled fertility, disease and inadequate education and infrastructure" (USAID

1990). Thus, USAID offered Tanzania a large package of aid to combat the problem of "uncontrolled fertility." USAID/Tanzania's "strategic objective number one" was "increased use of family planning, maternal and child health and HIV/AIDS preventive measures." The FPSS[27] budget that had initially committed $20 million over seven years, was increased to $30 million according to a 1995 report (Bureau of Statistics, Planning Commission, and The EVALUATION Project 1997, vi). By 1996, Tanzania had become the seventh largest recipient of 30 African countries receiving population assistance from the United States.[28] While population emphasis by USAID has declined in the 2000s, Tanzania remains one of the key programs where they continue to provide assistance.

The existence of a population policy was a crucial prerequisite for USAID commitment to family planning in Tanzania. A USAID project briefing states that "GOT [government of Tanzania] recognizes the serious economic impact of a high rate of population growth. In its population policy, GOT indicates it will use every available opportunity to control the growth of the population" (Mburu 1995, 8). The problem of population in the country is consistently recalled in discussions of the state of family planning in the country. The same project briefing notes the following two sentences that at first reading may appear to be nonsequiturs, but when taken in the larger political context serve to remind us of the underlying link between population and development in the discourse of donors. The document states:

In the words of President Mwinyi: "*The Government has a limited ability for becoming a successful entrepreneur due to a lack of resources.* The Government of Tanzania has a long way to go in controlling a runaway population growth" (Mburu 1995, 4, emphasis in original).

The implication here may be that the government has a lack of resources because it has not successfully controlled its population growth, or that a government that is poor must control its population growth. However, in these documents, the issue of the control of population growth (the goal) is spoken of as a development issue, while the issue of family planning (the means) is spoken of as a health issue. Perhaps it was politically expedient to disassociate family planning from population in the donor discourse to preclude any resurgence of the Bucharest criticisms (that rich countries are simply interested in reducing population in poor countries and have no real interest in health concerns). Indeed, part of what the donors gained in the Cairo consensus over reproductive health is a heightened ability to claim interest in larger health concerns.

Coordination of Various Interests

The FPU was established as a unit separate from the general MCH duties to ensure that family planning was promoted equally to other MCH components, such as prenatal care or child survival. This appears to have also served the function of allowing donors to more easily separate family planning from the other components. As described in the Country Report for the Third African Population Conference: "Monitoring and evaluation of the family planning activities from both government and NGOs is partly coordinated by the Family Planning Unit (FPU) in the Ministry of Health. Population IEC activities, including family planning, are coordinated by the Population Planning Unit of the Planning Commission in the President's Office while family planning service delivery is coordinated by the Ministry of Health" (United Nations Economic Commission for Africa 1992, 65). However, one "threat" noted in the "Structure and Management of the NFPP" is that "role demarcation and complementarity are unclear" between the family planning implementers and the population policy coordinators (United Republic of Tanzania 1994a, 7). In sum, family planning and population issues were being integrated more readily than family planning and other maternal and child health issues.

The UNFPA mid-term evaluation stated that strong collaboration between USAID and UNFPA had been an important factor in the NFPP success. While donor documents occasionally indicate that turf battles took place, the similarity in goals and objectives from one institution to another, as well as their willingness to collaborate in funding various components of the NFPP suggest that, whether or not they were well-coordinated, collaboration was taking place.[29] While the situation amongst policymakers and funders in Dar es Salaam was apparently somewhat clear from the beginning of the NFPP, there was little trickle down to implementers. The evaluation of the NFPP (1989–1993) asserts that "District and regional teams knew little or nothing about the National Family Planning Programme although they will be expected to implement it. There were no FP service plans" (Mpangile 1994, 64). This suggests the extent to which the NFPP was indeed a top-down operation, without much input even from the regional or district level personnel responsible for implementing it, much less the input of women who would be its targets. Through top-down projects requiring large expenditures, donors, in conjunction with development lenders, were directly and indirectly determining the discourse of family planning and pulling the strings of those responsible for implementing it.

UMATI (The Family Planning Association of Tanzania)

One of the most interesting implementing organizations is UMATI because it is the only local civil society organization with interests vested in family planning. If there is a particularly local official family planning discourse, or significant innovation within the national program, we would expect to see it in the workings of UMATI. Thus, this section examines UMATI's historical development and the next chapter examines one of its most local projects. With the changes brought about by the National Family Planning Programme and vast increases in donor funding, UMATI, which had historically been the only family planning organization, was called upon for the first time to justify itself. In 1996, UMATI was still the most significant NGO in Tanzanian family planning, and was often the only one mentioned when informants were asked about NGO participation in the family planning sector. For example, a USAID informant explained that there was "only one NGO in family planning—UMATI," but he went on to blame low family planning acceptance on their limitations: "UMATI's niche is in IEC [Information, Education and Communication], not in the provision of services which is why CPR [the contraceptive prevalence rate] has been very low."[30] The same informant told me in a follow-up interview: "In terms of outputs, you cannot compare UMATI with other clinics, or regional hospitals…it is not very significant."[31] UMATI's clinics themselves tend to be quite small, specialized, and located in urban areas. Since the beginning of government involvement and expansion of family planning in 1974, UMATI's role in service provision has been increasingly marginalized and its focus shifted.

However, UMATI is given credit for over 30 years of advocating for family planning at the local and national levels. A UNFPA representative stressed that UMATI gets credit for family planning success, through what can be described as the "barefoot doctor" approach, but that success also occurred because individual families have learned from bad experiences.[32] The World Bank also noted: "the present positive attitudes in the general public and various leadership levels are to a great extent attributed to UMATI" (Mpangile 1994, 9).

And indeed, UMATI itself took credit for bringing about the National Family Planning Programme, but recognized that this success has been bittersweet:

> Without question, it has been these pioneering efforts by UMATI that has led the Government of Tanzania to now publicly embrace a national Family planning policy and program. Now, however, UMATI is the victim of its own success. While previously, UMATI was largely able to define the family planning agenda for Tanzania, and thus its own strategy, it now appears somewhat overshadowed by the role of the public sector which has taken on the very areas in which UMATI has traditionally worked: contraceptive logistics, training of mid to lower level health workers, IEC, and most recently the establishment of community based delivery systems" (UMATI 1992, 2).

"A victim of its own success" indeed, starting with government involvement in family planning in 1974, but particularly since the inception of the national program, UMATI has been overshadowed by growing public sector involvement and donor diversification. Until 1990, UMATI was the sole institution providing training in basic family planning skills and had the responsibilities to procure, store, and distribute contraceptives and related commodities. However, after the government assumed these responsibilities, UMATI was forced to redefine itself.

One of UMATI's strengths, as perceived by international population donors, is its nongovernmental status. Some research in other areas has suggested that locally based NGOs function as grassroots organizations that are more connected with, and therefore more responsible to their constituents. Indeed, UMATI wisely promotes this interpretation by stressing that it is a *voluntary* organization, and its participants are referred to as "members," not clients. By the early 1990s, its membership was over 200,000 and its volunteer structure includes 800 branch committees, 83 district committees, 20 regional committees and a national executive committee (USAID 1990, 44). UMATI is dependent on foreign assistance for up to 96 percent of its budget, about 60 percent of which comes from IPPF (Mpangile 1994, 49). In 1990, USAID stated that approximately two-thirds of UMATI's annual $1 million budget comes from IPPF, with the rest coming from other donors (NORAD, SIDA, UNDP, JOICFP, and USAID) and membership dues (USAID 1990, 44). Bulatao (1993) argues that northern-based NGO's have a history of implementing the agenda of their funders, not of their clients. My research suggests that the agenda of funders is significant, regardless of the nature of the implementing organization.

With a heavy dependence on international aid money, UMATI was in a precarious position when the orientation of family planning was radically altered through the national program and when USAID became the major donor. USAID was known for being less lenient with its contractors than other donors, and UMATI had developed a reputation of being less efficient than some other organizations. A consultancy report elaborated the desired outcome between USAID and UMATI cooperation: "USAID-funded activities...will be quite specific in detailing the nature and content of the various activities and therefore, how the funds will be used. Policy and program decision making in the context of USAID funding will be a much less independent, autonomous exercise" (USAID 1990, 174). The report also called for UMATI to do comprehensive strategic planning, so that UMATI could demonstrate its usefulness in the new program.

At the same time, UMATI as an NGO was in a good position to take advantage of the American enthusiasm for private sector–led development. USAID promoted the private sector for service provision as a means of meeting demand in a cost effective way. The relationship between the supposed success of population programs and their reliance on the private sector is controversial. Bulatao argues that funds for population should be shifted from the state to the private sector, which, he claims, has the advantage of being more innovative, flexible, efficient, and linked to communities than the public sector (1993, 31–34). However, Mauldin and Ross (1989) argue that the data are inconclusive.[33] Despite the fact that the data available suggest that there is no reason to believe that NGOs will be inherently more participatory than their state counterparts, international donors in Tanzania are eager to fund NGOs in the family planning sector.

As UMATI's duties in family planning were being usurped by the state, the organization's focus was reoriented to accommodate demands that the government was less willing, or less equipped to meet. UMATI tried to refocus its direction into service delivery instead of a focus on demand generation (Mpangile 1994, 37). However, because of its extensive network of health facilitates and personnel, the government was in a stronger position to receive the influx of family planning aid money aimed at creating a national level program. The supposed "unmet demand" for family planning throughout the country meant that the lion's share of the program funding was on meeting the needs for contraception, rather than on programs to create more need. Therefore, UMATI could not claim its niche in either large-scale service provision, or in education as it had in the past. However, as an NGO with a handful of clinics and a network of members across the country, UMATI was in a prime position to take charge of a specialized and more controversial aspect of the national program—the permanent and long-term component.

UMATI assumed responsibility for projects initiated and supported by donors, which would not, at least initially, have been part of the national menu of family planning services. For example, the Ministry of Health designated UMATI as the implementing agency for permanent and long-term contraception in the country. This was the largest sub-project within USAID's family planning support, and by the mid-term review, it was expected to cost about $3,500,000 over the life of the project—over $2 million more than had been originally planned (USAID 1994, A-12). The project began in 1988, and by 1991, UMATI had trained 21 counselors and 14 minilaparotomy teams (doctor and nurse teams). UMATI began the introduction of Norplant® in October 1991 in two of its Dar es Salaam clinics. This was then expanded to UMATI clinics in Mbeya and Moshi. The project was not specifically designed to address Norplant, but when it was introduced in Tanzania it fit well within USAID's objectives of supporting long-term contraception. However the politics of long-term contraception and potential links to population coercion were never far below the surface. For example, during one day of participant observation in an UMATI urban clinic, I was alone in the waiting room with a client who had come in to see if she would be given Norplant. She had been to the clinic the week before and had been found to have high blood pressure, so she was told to wait a week and then return to check again. Immediately, she turned to me and asked, "Do you use these too, or do you just put them in us?" UMATI as a local institution was in the position to negotiate the politics of discontent between local recipients and international donors.

In describing their new strategic approach, UMATI reiterated:

> UMATI is no longer in the position of determining the shape and strategy of the national Family Planning program; that responsibility now appropriately rests with the government. Furthermore, the breadth and depth of the government health infrastructure will be to a large extent determine [*sic*] the predominant mode of service delivery. Thus, for UMATI to continue to make an important contribution to the national

> program, it will necessarily be through highly leveraged activities which will lead the national program into new areas, or to provide technical support on government run activities" (UMATI 1992, 3).

The activities where UMATI planned to make its contribution were: 1) introduction of long-term methods;[34] 2) coordination of private sector activities; 3) community based service delivery; and 4) establishment of services aimed at youth and young adults.[35] In what is clearly indeed a strategic approach, UMATI responded to the agenda of international donors by agreeing to implement projects in controversial areas (i.e., vasectomy promotion and targeting youth and unmarried women) and/or areas where UMATI was known for expertise that the government lacked (for example, community based service delivery). The risk was that UMATI was becoming known for promoting unpopular methods. A regional medical officer stated: "UMATI is advocating vasectomy nowadays, although people are against it. They are introducing it, but nobody volunteered."[36]

If UMATI was to continue to play a role in the national program, it had to work in cooperation with the government sector. Officially, my informants from both UMATI and the government said that relations were good between workers in the various sectors. For example, a district MCH coordinator explained that UMATI supplies contraceptives if government clinics run out; that is, in 1995 they ran out of Depo-Provera and got it from UMATI.[37] A regional coordinator stated: "Now we work with them [UMATI], especially for minilap and Norplant. We are sharing doctors. Also, if they need supplies, they can come over here, etc. We are working together on joint supervision as well."[38] Another district coordinator confirmed: "UMATI and MOH share training, health education, and CBD projects—the Primary Health Committees have a representative from UMATI." She went on to state that "the MOH has higher levels of knowledge and ability, so it was better to work together to increase their combined abilities."[39]

However, while the official stance was one of cooperation, conflicts between the government and UMATI became apparent during my participant observation. For example, one of the sites I visited to observe family planning supervision was not scoring very well on the family planning evaluation done by the government. The service provider in charge had been trained by UMATI, and as soon as it was clear that the evaluation was not going well, the district MCH coordinator quickly pointed out to the other members of the evaluation team that for a long time the clinic had not even been under the Ministry of Health. She claimed that she had not received any of the clinic reports; they went to UMATI. It was clear that they thought that UMATI was doing an inferior job of training and supplying their people, after finding two boxes of expired pills in the cabinet. The evaluation team advised the service provider to strengthen her relationship with the district coordinator from the government.[40] The government evaluators told the service provider: "UMATI can always pull out, but the government is always here."[41]

In this interaction, it was clear that the government representatives wanted to distance themselves from a clinic that was not meeting their supervision standards, and blaming UMATI was one way of doing this. Another example comes from a government family planning trainer who claimed the government family planning nurses are more motivated than those at UMATI and they have a better working situation in the public sector than with the NGOs because of more job security and government benefits.[42]

The perception that somehow UMATI is being favored by funders because it is given particular methods that the government does not supply, and that it is operating outside of the formal system, was elaborated by a regional medical officer. When I asked him about UMATI activities in his region, he replied: "It is not part of the government structure, so I don't know much about what they are doing."[43] He also had not heard that the Japanese Aid Organization was giving UMATI assistance, although after probing, he did say that he had heard vaguely of the Integrated Project (IP), which he referred to as "that project on deworming and distribution of family planning pills."[44] This project will be discussed in more detail in the next chapter.

While one of UMATI's challenges was to avoid conflict with the government, it was also confronted with a rapidly growing number of other NGOs in family planning—all of whom were competing for their share of donor money. A representative from one funding organization explained that their funding for "local NGOs" was no longer going to UMATI "because their performance was low and in family planning alone."[45] My informant elaborated that her organization gave assistance for UMATI CBD projects such as the family planning project at the UDSM; however, when the funder withdrew, the project collapsed and then they would not work through UMATI because of their problems.[46] These problems will be elaborated in the next chapter examining one of UMATI's flagship project, the Intergrated Project on Nutrition, Parasite Control and Family Planning.

The Success of Family Planning in Tanzania

In light of the complex historical context of the institutionalization of family planning services in the country as described so far, the successes of the National Family Planning Programme may come as a bit of a surprise. However, the family planning of health care has been reasonably successful in meeting the goals of increased awareness and use of modern contraceptives. The meaning and limitations of this success are points to which I return in the book's conclusions. In Tanzania today, contraceptives are usually provided within an integrated clinic structure designed for family planning and maternal and child health services. This clinic may be situated within different types of health care structures: 1) a dispensary, the smallest type of health facility designed to serve a ward with a population of about 6,000; 2) a health center, with 20–30 beds that is supposed to function as a small hospital; or 3) a hospital, which may be classified as district, regional or consulting (Bureau of Statistics, Planning Commission et al. 1997, 53). Private services are available for a fee from some church-based or NGO providers (such as the Marie Stopes or UMATI [the Tanzanian Family Planning Association]). Yet, three-fourths of all family planning users obtain their contraceptives from government sources (Ibid.), and more than 60 percent of all health services are provided by the government (National Bureau of Statistics et al., 2000). Thus, public service provision is still the most important source of Tanzania's reproductive health care. As described in chapter five, the state of the public health clinics seriously limits the quality of reproductive health care that can be provided.

Nonetheless, in spite of the potential limitations of an ambivalent policy, conflicting implementing agencies, and a health care structured dilapidated by years of a declining economy, Tanzania's National Family Planning Programme claims a striking level of "success" if policy implementation is assessed on the criterion of fertility reduction. As early as 1993, an independent consultant of USAID was reported to have said that "a miracle has been wrought" (United Nations Population Fund 1994, annex E). Family planning was offered in approximately 90 percent of Tanzanian health clinics by 1996. Between the early- and mid-1990s, Tanzanian family planning use nearly doubled, and continued to rise slightly at the end of the decade as shown in table 3.2.

Table 3.2 Current Use of Family Planning by Married Women

Source	*TDHS 1991/1992 (%)*	*TDHS 1996 (%)*	*TRCHS 1999 (%)*	*TDHS 2004/2005 (%)*
Any Method	10.4	18.4	25.4	26.4
Any Modern Method	6.6	13.3	16.9	20.0

Source: 1991/1992 and 1996 Tanzania Demographic and Health Surveys, 1999 Tanzania Reproductive and Child Health Survey, 2004/2005 Tanzania Demographic and Health Survey.

Knowledge of contraception is quite high (in 93.5 percent of all couples, both know a modern method of family planning according to the 1999 TRCHS). Trends in fertility preferences have shifted during the period of the 1990s and into the 2000s, with fewer married women wanting another child "soon" and more wanting no more children. Total fertility rates also declined from 6.5 in the 1988 census to 6.2 by the 1991/1992 DHS, 5.8 by the 1996 DHS and 5.6 by the 1999 TRCHS. Most recently, total fertility rates seem to have stabilized and were documented at 5.7 by the 2004/2005 DHS. We do not know how much of Tanzania's fertility decline can be attributed to increased contraceptive use. Another cause of lower fertility rates is infertility—higher in Tanzania than in neighbouring countries.[47] Furthermore, Lloyd, Kaufman, and Hewett (1999) argue that Tanzania still has lower levels of contraceptive use than expected when compared to other African countries with similar levels of educational attainment. However, it is not my point to assess the efficacy of the family planning program on fertility, but to point out that family planning has gone up at the same time as fertility has declined.

In conclusion, we know that the total fertility rate is dropping in Tanzania, as it is in many other parts of the developing world, even if it is not certain how much of the decline can be attributed to contracepting in general, or to the family planning program specifically. Without question, donors have succeeded in funding a national family planning program that has raised awareness, access, and use of contraceptives throughout the country.

However, Tanzania has been less successful in improving other aspects of reproductive health. For example, the proportion of births assisted by trained personnel has declined steadily, and women are less likely to receive professional assistance at delivery than they did in the 1970s (see Richey 2003). As late as my fieldwork in 2000, clinics were often lacking in essential supplies, including basic drugs. In addition, a nationally representative survey found that less than 1 percent of government dispensaries had a working light source, laboratory, or refrigerator (National Bureau of Statistics Tanzania, and MEASURE Evaluation 1999). Shortages of basic equipment and supplies in Tanzanian clinics is an ongoing problem (see also Rajani 2002). The success of contraceptive provision in light of such basic failures in other services presents a reproductive health paradox in Tanzania (Richey 2004). This paradox will play an important role in the potential for Tanzania's provision of reproductive health in the future, a point to which the book's conclusion will return.

Conclusion

Despite the ambivalence of the Tanzanian government over the role of family planning within the National Population Policy, the National Family Planning Programme has been, in effect, the implementation of that policy. Family planning for childspacing purposes initiated before the end of colonialism, and it continued with tacit government support throughout the early independence period. The Tanzanian government's commitment to family planning services was made explicit with its 1974 inclusion of childspacing as an important element of its larger program for women's and children's health. The time between the government's official involvement and the start of a national program in 1991 was characterized by negotiations between donors, lenders, and the government. The real interests and official positions of various actors were strategic and contextually specific. However, the dependence on foreign money for the lion's share of the funding in this area meant that the government and UMATI had limited power for negotiation over what kinds of interventions would constitute Tanzania's program.

A donor-constructed agenda taking a demographic approach for dealing with population is not unique to Tanzania, and in fact, remains common in Third World countries receiving population assistance. However, the Tanzanian government's historical emphasis on primary health care and avoidance of population control measures meant that the national program had to balance the desires of donors for population reduction with those of its constituents. The interplay of different perspectives on the population problem, women's reproductive health needs, and the authority to control fertility decision making continues from the policy discourses through the implementation forms and into local clinics and projects. The following chapters will analyze these projects and the local lenses through which the global population discourse is realized in Tanzanian communities. As this chapter has shown, the meaning of family planning, whether it refers to a general notion of childspacing by any means or to the adoption of modern contraceptive methods, is a political category as well as a personal action. Yet, as Tilly describes, "away from the boundary [of formed categories] plenty of room exists for gradations, ambiguities, and further classifications" (1999, 347). To make family planning acceptable in the face of local discontent over perceived population control ideologies, one long-running project linked contraceptive provision with other local development objectives. The following chapter describes the archetypal example of attempting to reconcile the demographic, development, and feminist narratives of the global population discourse in the practice of a donor-funded intervention.

4

Humanistic Family Planning—Governing Population at the Grassroots

Introduction: The Integrated Project and Holistic Interventions

If you ask donors for money for poverty, they say no, but if you ask for it for family planning, you will get it (Participant at the International Workshop on the Integrated Project).

The reproductive health agenda, like other neomodernization discourses of development progress, assumes that development, feminist, and demographic goals are synergistic. This "all good things go together" assumption is challenged when such wide-ranging projects are implemented in a local context of resource scarcity. The integrated approach toward family planning with development has a much longer history from which we can draw lessons. This chapter examines an NGO-run integrated family planning project in Tanzania to illustrate how competing agenda, embedded within a web of relationships—international donors, state, NGO, and local recipients—manifest themselves in implementation at the village level. The Integrated Project on Family Planning, Nutrition and Parasite Control, known as the "Integrated Project" has been operating in Tanzania for nearly two decades with the goals of integrating family planning service provision with projects that address other community needs.[1] The Integrated Project provided the foundation for contemporary interventions termed "community-operated integrated reproductive health approach" that now operate in 26 countries (Fukuda 2005). This approach is based on experience from the integrated projects, but framed in the post-Cairo language of reproductive and sexual health.

Field research in three Tanzanian Integrated Project villages, with the implementing family planning organization, and with the project's international donors reveal how goals of fertility reduction, local-level involvement, and women's empowerment are juxtaposed with issues of negotiating accountability, competition for economic spoils, and opportunist politics. A leader of this project reconciles the opposing goals of empowerment, demography, and sensitivity to local realities by constituting a new recipient, the "passive acceptor." This passive acceptor is at the intersection of meeting locally felt needs, depoliticizing gender, and showing success from a demographic perspective. The case of the Integrated Project demonstrates instances when what happens on the ground cannot simply be attributed to local culture or to state intervention, but also relates to a global discourse and agenda. Understanding the dynamics of competing agenda at the level of project implementation makes an important contribution to my analysis of the interface between global discourse and local politics.

The Integrated Project has been deemed a "more humanistic approach to family planning" (Urrio 1995, 28). Unlike other family planning projects that limit themselves to providing information and supplies of contraceptives, this project is based on a model of meeting community needs first, and providing family planning afterward. The deputy executive director of the project's international funder stated: "If we wish to persuade the inhabitants in the worst conditions to turn their attention to the importance of family planning, food production and medical campaigns, rather than family planning, should be given priority" (Curtis 1989, 3). Indeed, the principles of the project's philosophy were in the vanguard for promoting a larger agenda, which would come to be articulated in Cairo as women's reproductive health. In the project, family planning should be linked more closely with family health and welfare than with population control. "To this end, some other service beneficial and fundamental to daily life should be integrated with family planning, thus increasing the credibility of family planning workers" (International Planned Parenthood Federation [IPPF] 1988, 5).

This holistic approach toward family planning was portrayed as supporting the goals of the National Population Policy, while the policy itself provided an environment of greater political acceptability for the Integrated Project. A Tanzania country paper lists the goals of the National Population Policy that are particularly relevant to the objectives of the Integrated Project:

1. To achieve a *lower population growth rate* through reduction of birth rate by voluntary fertility regulation.
2. *Improve health and welfare for the population in general* through prevention of premature deaths and illness.
3. Promote equality of rights, opportunities and treatment in life and work for all Nationals with specific attention to *improving the status of women* (UMATI 1995a, 4, 5, emphasis added).

Here we see the national policy and the project as implementing three different agenda: 1) a demographic agenda—goals of fertility reduction and population control); 2) a development agenda—goals of local level involvement and improvements in the lives of villagers); and 3) a feminist agenda—concentrating specifically on the needs of women and their empowerment). As we have seen in the previous chapters, these agenda were not universally accepted in either the population policy circles or in family planning implementation. The following discussion will show how these agenda and the conflicts between them are seen in local level implementation through an examination of the integrated project.

The following section will examine a history of the integrated project as an example of community-based distribution of contraceptives. Then, the third section looks at the links between the various project components: what does deworming have to do with preventing babies? The next section looks at the integration aspects that are integral to the project's identity. Section five analyzes two controversial elements of the project, income-generating activities and incentives, arguing that these two can often become intertwined in practice. Then, the next three sections look in turn at different goals following from diverse global narratives: development, demographic, and feminist. The concluding section analyzes how the goals of the project, like the global narratives themselves, can find themselves at loggerheads with each other, challenging the notion underlying both reproductive health and neoliberal modernity that all good things go together.

History of the Integrated Project on Family Planning, Nutrition, and Parasite Control

The Integrated Project in Tanzania, initiated in 1984, was the first Integrated Project in Africa, and one of the longest running Community Based Distribution (CBD) projects in Tanzania. CBD projects use members of local communities to distribute contraceptive information and supplies. CBD projects are viewed by some as inherently more responsive to the needs of local communities because of their decentralized approach, which does not subject family planning clients to the often-disempowering medical environment of the clinic (Helzner and Shepard 1997). At the same time, CBDs are also considered to be a cost saving alternative means of demand creation and health care provision. According to USAID, "although the cost of CBD programs may be expensive up front, once solid demand is created and women (and men) understand that family planning is safe and effective, they will go far to obtain methods on their own. CBD programs can eventually be phased out or CBD agents can set up a depot for supplies and clients can come to them" (USAID 1994, 43). Thus, CBD projects are used to build up a client base, and then later phased out, without consideration of whether they provide a more empowering environment for clients.

The Integrated Project is one of many CBD projects in Tanzania.[2] Some CBD agents are paid project employees and others are volunteers. Each CBD program has its own objectives and guidelines, although all are supposed to conform to national protocols and use the same training and supervision tools.[3] The introduction to the revised National CBD Guidelines referred specifically to the post-Cairo shift in the discourse stating that "these guidelines strive to examine family planning as part of women's reproductive health" (Mpango wa Taifa wa Uzazi wa Mpango na Afya ya Uzazi 1997, iii).[4] Whether or not the CBD modality for providing contraceptives is actually better suited to the task of local translation of global discourse and technologies, it is a means of expanding the cadre of gatekeepers beyond the more professionalized cadre of formal health care.

The Integrated Project is administered through UMATI from its national office in Dar es Salaam, regional offices in each region of implementation, and local level supervisors. Each project site also has a Local Steering Committee that is supposed to act as the decision-making body at the local level; however, as I show later in the chapter, this is not often the case. The persons responsible for actually implementing the project in the villages are the CBDs. From the beginning, the project tries to create an identity for the CBDs that is modern and positive in ways that are similar to the formal service providers at the local clinics as I will discuss in the next chapter. These individuals represent an important link between the moral character of the agent and the legitimacy of the contraceptive methods and message. The criteria for selection of CBD agents include:

- Education: the person selected must be literate, he/she should be able to read and write at least Kiswahili, which is the national language.
- Influence in the community: the person selected should be an influential and respectful person in the community.
- The person should not be a close relative (daughter, son, nephew) of the community leader in that particular community. This is to avoid favoritism and other conflicts in the community (Urrio 1995, 19).

As the criteria above demonstrate, CBDs, should conform to the neoliberal ideal citizen—educated, respectable, and corruption-free, and are meant to provide a certain positive image of the project in their communities.

In 1983, two areas were selected as project sites for the initiation of the project: 1) Roo and Modio, in Masama ward in Hai District (population of approximately 10,000 people) and 2) the sugar plantation run by the Tanganyika Planting Company (TPC) in an enclosed camp setting in Arusha Chini (population of approximately 8,000 people). Both are located in Kilimanjaro Region, where we return in chapter six for more detail, an area known for high population density, the highest educational levels, and its modern identity. The reasons for choosing these two sites, out of all of the possible Tanzanian villages, are summed up in an official field visit report:

> The main advantages of Arusha Chini are the well-established medical system, including a hospital with good laboratory facilities that can be made available to the project, the right population density of 15,000 people,[5] easy accessibility of the area from Moshi and a very cooperative head of the medical establishment at TPC (IPPF 1988, 2).

This site was actually defined as "peri-urban," and enclosed in a parastatal sugar plantation. The same report describes Masama as "a typical rural area…The road to Masama is all-weather although not bitumized part of the way, and there is a health centre located in the village which offers a variety of facilities including a small laboratory" (IPPF 1988, 2). Of course, all-weather roads and health facilities with laboratories are anything but "typical" of Tanzanian villages.

A National Steering Committee was formed in 1983 with representatives from UMATI, the Ministry of Health, and Muhimbili Medical Centre. In spite of the use of "nutrition" in the title, a project review noted that "no nutritionist was included; it was felt that special nutrition studies would not be necessary because children who have been de-wormed are manifestly much more healthy than before" (IPPF 1988, 21). From its inception, the components of what was supposed to be an integrated project received varying degrees of emphasis.

The project began by putting forth its parasite control component in an attempt to meet a "felt need" of the communities. Once trust was gained by the project, then family planning messages and supplies would be distributed. In 1984, the project began in Kilimanjaro with a mass stool examination and blanket treatment of all adults and children in the project areas. A project evaluation noted that at this time "Family planning education is fully integrated with education about sanitation and nutrition, usually delivered through health education talks and films complemented by home visits" (IPPF 1988, 22). Early on, the project experienced leadership difficulties with the resignation of the project director and termination of contracts of two other senior staff.[6] Nevertheless, "a 1988 evaluation of the project found that the project has achieved recommendable mobilisation and increase in awareness in environmental hygiene and family planning practice" (Urrio 1995, 4). Once the project was in full swing, it began expanding to other villages and other regions of the country.[7]

During the initial phases of introducing the project into new villages, the CBDs met with local resistance. One informant said that when the project began distributing contraceptives and providing family planning education, a local priest told parishioners that the UMATI people had no business in the village and that if they saw any of the CBDs, they "should throw stones at them." The conflict peaked when one CBD was actually hit and had to be taken to the hospital. Soon afterward the priest was transferred to another area, and his replacement was more tolerant of family planning.[8] In another village, CBDs described how the entire first year of the project was difficult because UMATI had a bad name in the village and local people were afraid of them. One CBD explained that in the beginning, her neighbors would hide and pretend that they were not at home when she came around in her role as a CBD.[9]

CBDs related that the initial projects were difficult to implement, but once the word got out, and they went to villages that had requested the project, things went more smoothly. Informants stated that villages near but not included in the project asked for it to be expanded into their territory. When the project was being initiated into a new site, a baseline survey was conducted by UMATI, and then regional, district, and local leaders, along with members of the community where the project would be, were sensitized. During sensitization, recipients "are introduced to the National Population Policy and the Demographic situation of the country, economic and social status of the country and support/stand of the government on family planning services (Urrio 1995, 24). At the same time that sensitization focuses on promoting family planning as a response to overpopulation, the integrated project's supposed innovation is not its family planning component, but successful integration of family planning into other development aspects such as parasite control, nutrition, and income generation.

Parasite Control, Nutrition, and Family Planning: What does Deworming have to do with Preventing Babies?

In the early stages some school children were prevented from receiving treatment by parents who associated it with the family planning service and were afraid that their children might get sterilized (IPPF 1988, 27).

Worms were the legitimating entry point into local communities, but lost emphasis as donor-prioritized family planning became less controversial. The description of the integrated project in UMATI's 1996–1998 Three Year Plan emphasizes how "through showing concern of [*sic*] an immediate health problem (worms) as perceived by the communities, the project staff manage to boost their personal images and create appropriate rapport that then becomes instrumental in ensuring project success" (UMATI 1996, 43, 44). Therefore, a prerequisite for an integrated project site is that it must be an area with a high prevalence of soil transmitted intestinal worms (Urrio 1995, 5). Ascariasis was the worm of choice in Kilimanjaro and Morogoro Regions, but as it was rare in Mwanza, the project instead took on the more common hookworm.

In the initial phases of the project in Kilimanjaro Region, mass stool examination and subsequent deworming were carried out in 1985 in TPC and again in 1987 in Masama. According to an evaluation report, "selective treatment twice a year was adopted, together with provision for treating individuals on request" (IPPF 1988, 27). There was initial resistance to the deworming; as noted in project documentation, "[t]he association between family planning and worms has not been easily understood. Consequently, some parents refuse to allow their children to take antihelmithics offered through family planning systems construing them to be contraceptives" (Urrio 1995, 9). Yet the demonstrable success of the treatment converted those who were initially skeptical, as indicated by the introductory remark:

> However these parents became more confident when the effects of deworming began to be visible. A powerful illustration of these effects was provided by the fact that after mass treatment at TPC [Tanganyika Planting Company], communal drains were sometimes blocked with worms (IPPF 1988, 27).

As planned, the effectiveness of the deworming led credibility to the project and its workers who could then convert this legitimacy toward promoting family planning.

As the project advanced, stool examinations were to be conducted in the primary schools, with mass dewormings done at 6-month intervals (UMATI 1995a, 8). However, UMATI data show deworming done at the Bati site in Morogoro Region show at intervals of 12 months, 6 months, and even 18 months (UMATI 1995a, 9). UMATI expressed dissatisfaction with the continuing high levels of worm infestation, and placed the blame on the communities themselves. The "likely" reason given by UMATI for why the prevalence continued to be high was that "de-worming is the only method at work. The communities have not yet changed their behaviours relevant to worm infections and high rates of latrinization are notwithstanding" (UMATI 1995a, 9). The UMATI report continues that "villagers do not understand the association between family planning and worms," so they refuse to participate in the deworming (Ibid.). When the deworming was taking place regularly and results were visible in the communal drains, the project assumed credit for the success, but when positive results were less forthcoming, the project's recipients were held responsible for thwarting the goals through their incorrect behavior and lack of understanding. In a discussion of constraints, the project report acknowledges that "for logistic and other reasons, it has not been possible to follow the de-worming schedules to the letter and this may have also contributed to the relatively slow drop in prevalence rates over the years" (UMATI 1995a, 10).

A situation analysis comparing project villages in Morogoro and Kilimanjaro Regions with a comparable non-project village found that the prevalence of helminthic infestations among children under five was *higher* in project areas than in non-project areas (Tanzania Food and Nutrition Centre 1995, 41).[10] While it may indeed have been the case that communities were reticent in their participation, it is also likely that the parasite control component was not being emphasized because it was becoming increasingly less useful for showing success in the demographically oriented components of the project. Furthermore, the demographic goals of the project were fueling local fears and rumors of involuntary sterilization.

The deworming component clearly lost momentum as time went on. During interviews, CBDs explained that they conducted community education about worms and larger issues of sanitation, but that the actual deworming was done only sporadically because of lack of medicines. In fact, during my participant observation and interviews with participants in three project villages, the only sign of deworming I encountered was a lengthy intestinal worm in formaldehyde kept in a jar on the desk of the regional project supervisor. When I asked about the worm, the supervisor told me that it had come from a child during their deworming in schools. The fact that a worm had come from the intestines of a village child to the jar on a project desk speaks the need to "show" in tangible, physical, and measurable terms, what the project was accomplishing. The worm in itself was at once a representative of how the project was responding to the "felt needs" of villagers, and of how "evidence" had to be given of project success. Of course, a single worm, like a smattering of statistics, says nothing about reliability, continuity, or accountability of the project.

An informant, formerly with UMATI, explained: "When the IP began it went well. They did the stool exams and de-worming regularly, but then after a while, there was a problem with too few staff and funds for medicine for de-worming."[11] By the 1996–1998 Three Year Plan, UMATI states that while deworming would be done "more systematically" than in the past, the drugs for treatment would be sold at cost, instead of given to participants free of charge (UMATI

1996, 45). Selling the drugs, even at subsidized prices, would most likely exclude many of the project's intended recipients, especially the poorest members of the village. Once it was no longer needed as an entry point into communities, deworming remained in descriptions and justifications of the project but did very little in practice. A doctor involved in a different community health program that overlapped with the integrated project in some villages said that the number tested and dewormed was too small to have any impact in the villages.[12]

When the parasite component was no longer essential for legitimating the project, it lost out to other aspects competing for project funding and attention. However, the project could not simply drop the parasite control component. As a companion project to family planning, it served the symbolic role of showing that UMATI was addressing the felt needs of the community, indicated by the worm in formaldehyde. Since the integrated project was in no danger of losing donor support on the basis of a poorly performing helminth control program, but would be threatened by a poorly performing birth control program, UMATI wisely concentrated its means accordingly. This resulted in resources being spread too thinly to have had a sustained impact on parasite control.

The nutrition component faced difficulties comparable to those in the parasite control projects: nutrition was symbolically important, but received little priority in implementation. The Tanzania Food and Nutrition Centre noted that the project activities dedicated to nutrition were "very limited" and involved only "garden demonstrations and promoting consumption of locally available nutritious food" (Tanzania Food and Nutrition Centre 1995, 50).

In contrast to the nutrition and parasite components, the family planning component became more central after UMATI's 1993 Strategic Plan that changed the project's focus from raising awareness of family planning through sensitization to "effective contraceptive service delivery."[13] Thus, after 1993 the main functions of CBDs were to make home visits to deliver contraceptives and to counsel and make referrals for clients desiring a longer-term method. In one village, UMATI even had a car to transport clients to its urban clinic to receive long-term and permanent contraception.[14] While the project title and philosophy suggests an integrated project, the actual integration of non-family planning components proved limited. Still, these *other* aspects differentiated the project from more narrowly defined family planning projects, and provided proof of UMATI's status as a grassroots organization.

How Integrated is the "Integrated Project"?

We are in the business of family planning and this should not be lost sight of! (Participant at the International Workshop on the Integrated Project).[15]

The idea of an integrated project that, in addition to providing contraceptives it also funds projects aimed at meeting other development needs is a timely approach to family planning, and one which suits the Tanzanian context. The philosophy of integration fits very well into the post-Cairo discourse of expanding family planning to include a much broader field of women's reproductive health, which also has a strong economic component. Poor women are not healthy women. The integration philosophy also fits within the implementation strategy of the national policy. One government official brought up the integrated project as a positive example. He explained that "the JOICFP project is very nice...if they package [family planning] it can be taken anywhere; you can identify the local problems...if it's so dry, then no one can accept it."[16] However, my research suggests that the level of actual integration of non-family planning components is limited for nutrition and parasite control, and ambiguous for income-generating activities. Still, it is the other aspects of the integrated project that differentiated it from narrowly defined family planning projects; therefore, income generation holds an important symbolic position in promotion of the project.

An area service delivery manager for UMATI told me: "Family planning is the last thing you talk of...it's a by the way thing...a passenger project."[17] However, statements made about the project by non-UMATI respondents called this into question. A doctor who worked in a community health project in one area where the project operates said, regarding the "integrated" nature of the project, "people feel it is a front for only family planning."[18] This is significant because it suggests that while the project is promoting the notion of implementing non-family planning development projects, either these projects are not significant enough to be considered central to the integrated project, or UMATI's reputation with family planning is so entrenched that people assume that if UMATI is doing it, it must be family planning. Both factors likely explain why the project is sometimes seen as a front for family planning. In another instance, a village chairman of one project village told another researcher that he had *no idea* what the UMATI project did in his village.[19] Here, none of the project components made a significant impact on a village-level leader's perceptions. While this would seem at first to reflect negatively on the integrated project, it may represent a consciously strategic result, allowing UMATI to introduce a controversial project, family planning, in a way that does not bring undue attention to itself. However, it calls into question the level of involvement of village leadership in the integrated project and claims of "community responsiveness" at the local level.

An informant responsible for project implementation at the village level made clear that in the beginning of the integrated project in a particular area, donors wanted to do only family planning and not parasite control. My informant told how two representatives from the project's international donor had come to their village, and people asked them whether they would fund anything more than the family planning component. The donors were skeptical. As the informant related, "Finally, they were convinced to use parasite control as an entry point for family planning services."[20] To what extent the local communities actually had to convince donors to continue integrating the project cannot be substantiated. However, because the integrated project priorities shifted over time to increased emphasis on demographic goals, it is possible that donors wanted to cut out the parasite control component altogether. It is also interesting that while the official philosophy of the integrated project is to focus on meeting development needs and therefore humanizing family planning, the perceptions of the project on the ground are quite different.

If the development projects are simply a front for family planning, it is also the case that family planning is a way of bringing in donor money for development projects. During a group discussion at PANFRICO V, one participant suggested that "the 'humanistic approach' concept came from offering something more than just family planning." The integrated project also brings a means for local people to gain access to some project resources. UMATI-supplied bicycles get frequent use, and villagers are able to collect payments for time spent attending project meetings and training sessions. Also, some CBDs were making their own individual profit, both officially and surreptitiously, from various income-generating activities that were supplied by the project.[21] While these spin-offs may not be the intended development benefits, they are a way of bringing resources into villages. Also, women and men in project villages clearly have greater access to the contraceptives offered by the CBDs, making family planning more easily available for those who want it. The relationship between the diverse goals of the project is often ambivalent. Some agenda are used to justify others, while still competing with them for part of the project's budget.

My research suggests that this discrepancy between stated goals and actual implementation results from the attempt by the project to promote conflicting agenda. Which aspects of the project actually are emphasized is determined by the kinds of resources made available. These decisions are not made by local level project participants, nor by the national implementing agency (UMATI), but are ultimately in the hands of the project's funders. The difficulties of implementing these aspects of the project that make it a humanistic approach, that is, the development components, are well understood by project implementers. The integrated project is ultimately a family planning project, and thus, the demographic agenda—showing an increase in the use of contraceptives—takes precedence over responding to the perceived needs of the community. In a group discussion around the theme of humanistic family planning at an international conference, a participant noted that "you have to consider the community priorities and also your own resources; sometimes if you are given all of the needs, you won't do any family planning at all [for lack of enough resources]."[22] When implementers need to show "success," measured by how well they are meeting the demographic goals, for funding to continue, the development and feminist goals get marginalized.

Income-Generating Activities and Incentives in a "Voluntary" Project

Income-generating activities have an important, if ambiguous role in the implementation of the integrated project in rural villages. Income-generating activities are popular means of supporting small-scale economic ventures intended to help marginal groups begin the process of successful market integration. However, Patricia Stamp's work on gender and technology in Africa argues that such activities are "of questionable value or are even harmful to women" as they trivialize women's main work as food producers and reinforce "home economics" stereotypes that are popular within WID [Women in Development] approaches" (Stamp 1990, 50, see also Vavrus and Richey 2003). Nonetheless, income-generating activities are part of the integrated project and are meant to serve three different and potentially competing objectives. First, income-generating activities are held up as examples of how well the project is responding to local felt needs by providing useful projects as defined by these needs, such as milling machines or tractors. Second, access to "seed money" from donors is used to encourage villagers to participate in the Integrated Project. Third, income-generating activities have been discussed as a way of raising money for implementing other activities of the project to reduce dependence on donor funding.

Including income-generating activities is one way that the project can claim to be responsive to the needs of the villages where it is situated. Upunda (1995, 4) claims that "income generating groups are initiated by members of the community," but in my fieldwork, these bottom-up initiatives were preceded by extensive top-down facilitation. For example, in order to facilitate the initiation of income-generating activities under the integrated project in one village, a "lesson" [*masomo*] was given by an UMATI clinic director to an annual meeting of the Local Steering Committee. I was an observer at this meeting and was able to take notes on the lesson like the other participants. The first part of the lesson addressed the question as written in large handwriting at the front of the room: "Why do we need IGAs?" First, the director explained, that if donors withdraw, they can still continue the project. He drew a lengthy analogy with the Biblical reference "don't give a person a fish—teach him to fish."[23] This lesson was followed by a surprisingly technical discussion about how to perform double-entry bookkeeping. He elaborated that "our main goal is that afterward we will be able to provide services to our society. If you give someone money, then they think it is just a job and will quit if you stop paying them. This is why the IP is a voluntary project."[24] The second related explanation given as part of the lesson was that "in all countries, it is not the specialists who develop the country—it is voluntary action. If the young people see the way to lead a project, they will serve as role models for others in the village. The other main aim of the project is to serve as an example for others on how to develop."[25] Here, we have the emphasis on income-generating activities as development projects to "set examples" in the villages. We also see a high-level project administrator from town trying to "educate" local people about the meaning of "development from below." Symbolically, the Biblical reference, double-entry bookkeeping, and self-reliance provide a remarkable articulation of trying to inculcate "the villagers" with the trappings of neoliberal modernity. Family planning, added to development, would put everyone onto modernity's path, a far more worthy goal in the village context than simply distributing contraceptive pills.

A description of Tanzania's integrated project, lists the following roles for income-generating activities:

- To raise the economic status of community, which will enable them to decide and thus making family planning service delivery possible.
- To create avenues for women and men to meet and talk about FP, and provide themselves with FP methods.
- To strengthen volunteerism and team in order to strengthen FP service delivery and income generation.
- To generate income for sustainability of service provision (Urrio 1995, 17).

Three fourths of the roles for income-generating activities are about family planning, linking the development with the demographic goals. The first and last of these are interesting because they represent two potentially conflicting interpretations of the income-generating activities: "To raise the economic status of the community" implies that the income that is supposed to be generated from the project, belongs to the community. No clarification is given as to which members of the community will control this money—is it the participants specifically, integrated project participants as a whole, or the village or ward where the project takes place? It is also unclear if the money is to be held by individuals or groups, women, or men. If feminist goals are to be promoted, the gendered nature of control over resources must be taken into account, but it is not. The last role of income-generating activities—"To generate income for sustainability of service provision"—implies that any income will be reinvested in "service provision," understood to mean the provision of contraceptives, the only services provided. If this is the case, the activities are simply a way to raise local money to indirectly support the family planning component of the project.

The income-generating activities of the integrated project were similarly described by another long-time implementer in a different region. She said that first, UMATI provides motivation. Then, they give materials such as seeds or sewing machines. These projects are supposed to work at the individual level to "set examples" and at the ward level to "bring the CBDs together and give them some money."[26] Here the notion of the IGAs as providing incentives by offering some financial gain is emphasized. An UMATI report suggests that incentives were important for ensuring continued participation in the project noting that "by the end of the year all the 30 CBDs and all the young volunteers and TBAs were still with the project. This was made possible through the continued support they received from the project in terms of bicycles, materials for constructing the UMATI office, materials for the construction of the Guest House and for the clinic/pharmacy and the seed money for the afforestation programme" (Mkini 1995, 19).

However, in interviews with CBDs, it became clear that the integrated project was not meeting their expectations in the area of income generation. For example, when I asked about the activities involved in the project other than contraceptive distribution and health education, I was told by CBDs that there were "no other important things, only small activities from which they did not get much."[27] One CBD spoke up and said that none of these were making any profit. The rest of the group agreed, and went on to explain the failure of numerous projects: all but two pigs from the piggery project had died. Half of the mosquito nets they made remained unsold. Most of the saplings from the afforestation project died, and they had been able to sell only a few of the saplings that survived. The field that they had rented to farm a cash crop was also a failure. This left them with the selling of cloth, a pottery project, and a nursery school, about which they had no complaints. But at a later meeting I learned that the nursery school teacher had left because they had not been able to obtain enough money to pay the teacher's salary, and they had not been able to recruit another one.[28]

Most descriptions of income-generating activities link individual or communal financial gains from the activities to increasing levels of community development. This, of course, assumes that the projects will generate income, and that the management of these projects at the local level will be effective. There has also been a shift in the expectations over how any income will be spent. An agenda of reinvesting gains into the family planning component of the project is mentioned in discussions of project sustainability. Similarly, an UMATI paper stated: "the income generated from IGA, should be considered as sources of funds for purchase of contraceptives in future" (UMATI 1995a, 29). This new sustainability focus that potentially conflicts with community development goals suggests a need for local level implementers to show donors that there is community will to sustain the integrated project after donor money pulls out. In a framework more commonly associated with loans, projects must show they need money now, but will not need it indefinitely to carry out the same objectives. The idea of reinvesting local money into procuring supplies existed only in project documents and speeches to donors. It is unlikely that this sort of a change would be attempted, much less successful.

The fact that the integrated project is a voluntary project is symbolically important in establishing the legitimacy of its work. The reasoning is that if people participate voluntarily in the project, then it must be responding to their needs. However, the meaning of participation becomes more complex when we consider the issue of incentives. Some of the CBD programs in Tanzania pay their agents, while others are voluntary and thus rely on some form of incentive to encourage participation. There is no consensus on which approach is more effective, but having projects with different incentive or payment schemes can lead to conflict when some groups feel that others are receiving higher compensation for the same job.[29] The deputy director of the National Family Planning Programme noted that "existing differences about incentives to CBDs ought to be looked into further so that a common standard is followed" (UMATI 1995b, 16). When I asked a representative from USAID for his perspective on using incentives in CBD programs, he summed up his stance: "Paid workers work."[30]

Yet, the notion of UMATI as a voluntary organization is a foundational element of its institutional identity, and one that distinguishes it from the largest provider of family planning services, the Tanzanian government. Therefore, participants in the integrated project—CBD agents, Traditional Birth Attendants (TBAs), and Local Steering Committee members—all work on a voluntary basis. This is an important aspect of the project because it is a way that UMATI can claim that communities are eager to participate because they value the benefits so much that they do not need to be paid. However, a description of Tanzania's integrated project lists the following constraints and problems for CBDs:

- Strong will in doing something on a voluntary basis still lacks in Tanzania especially in areas where the project does not integrate other elements whose results can easily be seen.
- There are still small pockets of non-support which exist at village, ward and district levels.
- The spirit of ownership of the project at all levels is still weak.
- Work load for the CBD agents is too high for voluntary work e.g. providing services to more than 100 households (Urrio 1995, 22).

Many of these problematize the notion of an appropriate voluntary project. However, the way to overcome reticence among villagers is to offer them incentives. An UMATI report demonstrates the blurring of distinctions between incentives and payment: "Incentives to community based distribution of service agents should necessarily not be in monetary form. It should be in form of recognition of the good work performed and where possible support in the form of refresher courses to give them more technology in service provision" (Urrio 1995, 27). It goes on to note that "Incentives given in kind (e.g., sewing machines) enable the CBD agents to generate funds *for improvement of their families' health and for sustainability of the project*" (Ibid., emphasis added). There is an ambiguity over what the funds are to be used for: does "improvement of their families' health" mean that they will keep the money and use it to benefit their own families' health, or does it mean that because the integrated project is supposed to have health benefits, simply continuing the project would improve their families' health? Similarly, does "sustainability of the project" mean that the money raised by the integrated project will be reinvested in it, as discussed in the section on income-generating activities, or does it mean that by giving incentives, the project retains its CBDs and thus continues to operate?

The distinction between voluntary work and paid employment is blurred when the issue of incentives is taken into account. While project workers are unpaid, they do receive ongoing incentives for their participation in the project. Incentives come in the way of commodities and cash payment for attendance at meetings and training sessions. CBDs told me that they take a three-week course upon beginning the project, and each year they get a two-day refresher course. I was told by the leader of the CBDs in one village that each CBD had received a bicycle, rainboots, briefcase, a box for storing the contraceptives, and an umbrella.[31] These are not formally incentives, but, according to a report, are "participants' working tools"; they include the items previously mentioned as well as small pocket diaries, pens and pencils, hard cover register books, exercise books, and shoes (Mosha 1994, 8). The importance of these incentives was noted even in a report from one of the workshops acknowledging: "Participants' travel arrangements were good and they were pleased about the attractive amount of their per diem and commodities (working tools) given to them on the closing day of the workshop" (Mosha 1994, 7). The commodities' value is symbolic as well as material, as they act as identity artifacts designating modern service providers and bringers of development.

However, the provision of these artifacts as signs of belonging to a select group of affiliates created the expected conflict over project spoils. For example, UMATI documented one of the "implementation snags" as "lack of incentives to LSC [Local Steering Committee] members e.g. bicycles or motor cycles" (UMATI 1995b, 19). While bicycles can easily be understood as working tools for CBDs who must travel from house to house, it is harder to understand why members of the Local Steering Committee would need project-supplied transportation, and no explanation was given in the report. Members of the Local Steering Committee are paid a per diem and given food for the days when they attend UMATI meetings.[32] Not surprisingly, there is competition between participants over access to the incentives.

While incentives provide the basis for UMATI to maintain its authority in local-level implementation, the provision of incentives is difficult to negotiate. Incentives are supposed to be given to help CBDs in their work providing contraceptives, which can be relatively easily defined. However, they are also used to provide motivation, seed money, and compensation for time and money lost when attending project functions. Here the line between incentives as working tools and incentives as direct payment for participation in the project becomes quite blurred. I am not arguing that rural people should not be paid for providing services to their community; on the contrary, quite valid arguments can be made in favor of paying CBDs in the same way that other health care providers are paid.

However, my fieldwork suggests that incentives used in the CBD program are political tools used to ensure patronage and compliance, rather than payment for community health services. The use of incentives rather than payment for workers in the integrated project is used to maintain the image of UMATI as a voluntary organization, thus distinguishing it from the Tanzanian government. Incentives in kind are more difficult to compare directly from one village to another, so the lack of standardization allows more room for UMATI to use its own discretion in dispensing rewards. One informant noted that these incentives have also provided a problem for maintaining UMATI's credibility as a transparent, corruption-free organization. He described how the integrated project "gave out money, soap, fertilizer, and such as incentives. When these things remained after the meetings, the UMATI people themselves used the extra."[33] This was questionable behavior according to my informant, who feared that it might be seen as a kind of corruption. Furthermore, incentives are dependent on donations and thus are sporadic and changeable according to the project implementers. Many of them, such as the bicycles and UMATI uniforms, remain officially project property and are not actually given as property to individuals, so they can be revoked if a participant is not doing his or her job properly. Materially, the use of incentives, supplied by donors but controlled and distributed by UMATI, has the indirect result of increasing UMATI's legitimacy and prestige in local communities where it can be looked upon as a benefactor. Symbolically, these commodities, or working tools, are more than just small consumer goods, but also serve as identity artifacts for the UMATI participants. The kinds of items themselves are symbols of education (pens, notebooks, briefcases), mobility (bicycles, motorcycles) and hygienic discipline and modern style (shoes and umbrellas) (see Burke 1996, Ferguson 1999).

Participation: Local Level Involvement and "Development Goals"

Addressing socioeconomic concerns and local-level involvement are part of the development goals, linking family planning with other felt needs, both reproductive and productive. The regional director of the project's international donor described what he termed the "noble and humanistic approach" of the integrated project:

> Another commendable thing in the way the IP is normally implemented is the inclusion of poverty alleviation through the consideration of income generating activities that are designed and implemented again with the involvement of the beneficiaries, the implementing agencies and the Donors who provide seed resources. Poverty alleviation provides for a basis to look beyond the immediate reproductive health needs of the person at the centre of our activities (Okunnu 1995, 2).

The ways in which the integrated project embraces a development agenda are shown in three areas: design of the project that responds to locally felt needs, close links between project administrators and local people, and control of the project at the local level by the Local Steering Committee. The keynote speech at an Integrated Project conference elaborated the importance of socioeconomic development issues in the integrated project:

> When asked to identify their priority problems communities often mention water, malnutrition, poverty and diseases. IP in Tanzania is handling these problems in an integrated manner using the IP approach. In this way IP addresses not only the health problems of the people but also the socio-economic development of the people (Upunda 1995, 4).

Local involvement is one part of the Integrated Project's development goals. This agenda is ostensibly designed to motivate lethargic communities to accept the project and in the process, family planning. To the extent that the development agenda materially benefits women participants, it contributes to meeting their practical gender needs and thus, enhances this aspect of their empowerment. However, as I show below, these development goals also conflicted with feminist goals.

The project has capitalized on its community-based status and supposed responsiveness to local community needs. Initially, the project administrators actually lived in the rural project areas, which was a dramatic break from the usual way that such projects are run from afar. A 1988 evaluation report claimed this geographical proximity of leadership as "a turning point in the development of the project" (IPPF 1988, 25). In addition, the project is run in each village by the Local Steering Committee that supposedly operates by consensus (Urrio 1995, 29). In practice, relations between the village Local Steering Committee, the CBDs, and UMATI have been less than democratic. In the field, I discovered that important decisions were usually made in UMATI head offices, with local communities only informed later. For example, when project supervision was shifted back to town, and a new project supervisor introduced, the local CBDs were only informed when they witnessed the long-time supervisor packing up his belongings to leave his house in the village.[34]

I attended a Local Steering Committee meeting in one of the project villages[35] that was supposed to "clarify the UMATI charter and review their goals," but inadvertently reinforced the project hierarchy, with rural women at the bottom.[36] The manager of the UMATI clinic in town directed the meeting. He had driven to the village with a trainer, and the outgoing and incoming local project supervisors. The Local Steering Committee included all the important "big men" of the village—the ward secretary, the village chairman, the village health officer, the village extension officer, the doctor incharge of the rural health center—and two of the most active young female CBD agents. The clinic manager's dress, mannerisms, and language reinforced the class divide between himself and the villagers. During the meeting, he often "accidentally" spoke words in English, then struggled to translate them into Swahili. He spoke to the committee gently, but firmly, using the mannerisms of a primary school teacher. Still, he carefully insisted that everything must be decided by consensus. Yet, the power dynamic reinforced the role of the UMATI people from town as "experts," who could access resources for the elder committee members.[37] The CBDs, the only two rural women present, filled the roles of workers and helpers. During question and answer period of the lesson, the UMATI delegation called on the CBDs to give the anticipated "right" answer, but never did this to the elder men. At lunch, the CBDs served everyone else with food they appeared to have prepared themselves.

Interestingly, the two female members of the urban UMATI delegation spoke condescendingly to the CBDs, as if it were important to distinguish themselves as urban, educated, and salaried women. Women who had power as experts thus distanced themselves from the local women they were supposed to empower.[38] The development agenda of the Integrated Project is, in theory, what distinguishes it in theory from other family planning projects focused solely on contraception. However, as we have seen, participation on the ground is often either minimal or driven by a desire for individual gain. Moreover, if the development focus is no longer needed to attract family planning clients, its priority declines.

Demographic Goals: Promotion of Permanent and Long-Term Contraception

In the post-Cairo environment, the project's demographic agenda has become implicit rather than explicit. However, increasing contraceptive use in order to reduce population growth has remained the driving force behind the project. For example, UMATI's 1993–1995 Three Year Plan claims the project is "recording an increasing demand for long acting (e.g., Depo-Provera and IUDs) and permanent methods of contraception," and thus assisting in population reduction (UMATI 1993, 19, 20). The 1996–1998 Plan reiterates this theme (UMATI 1996, 45). The emphasis is on "long acting and permanent methods" that will reduce fertility rates more effectively than the condoms, foam, or pills distributed by CBDs.

UMATI's 1996–1998 Three Year Plan expects "60–70 percent of clients contacted by the project's CBD agents will opt for voluntary sterilizations, Norplant, Depo-Provera and IUDs' by 1998" (UMATI 1996: 45). This estimate makes little sense in a country where fewer than 12 percent of women opted to use modern contraception (Bureau of Statistics 1997a). This figure suggests a need to demonstrate success no matter how improbable.

In one project village, CBDs believed incentives were being offered for agents referring women for sterilization.[39] I heard a CBD group leader inform an agent that she would get a gift [*zawadi*] for every five sterilization referrals. During an interview with all the CBDs, the leader reluctantly admitted that he had had just "heard" this and maybe no one else knew. One person dared to agree with him. They all agreed the gift was only for sterilization. Informally I learned that the "gift" was 5,000 Shillings [approximately $8.50], a considerable amount of money in local terms. While I could not substantiate this rumor, it is important that the CBD agents believed it. This also demonstrates their belief that reducing fertility is an important part of the integrated project's goals.

The integrated project must be understood within the international demographic narratives emphasizing fertility reduction and the national politics of family planning service provision. The focus on Permanent and Long-Term contraception reflects UMATI's struggle to redefine itself in a newly competitive field of family planning, as described earlier in chapter three. By promoting the demographic goal of population reduction, UMATI has positioned itself as a complement to government service provision. Demographic goals have been highlighted to prove that UMATI can provide controversial services and remain linked to local communities. However, the consequences for women who are offered sterilization raise issues about voluntary choice in family planning. Local fears of an underlying population control agenda as described earlier in this chapter are fueled by improvisation by local CBDs to ensure project success.

The Feminist Agenda: Depoliticizing Gender and "Passive Acceptors"

> *These UMATI people and their money…those women don't know anything. They're just farmers and they are getting chai ["tea"—idiomatic use meaning "money"] all the time!*[40]

As discussed in chapter one, shifting narratives in the international arena changed the global population discourse after the 1994 Cairo Conference, and feminist narratives took a place alongside the long-touted demographic and development narratives. Integrated project implementers at the local level placed demographic goals alongside less promoted, but rhetorically important, feminist demands for improved gender relations and women's empowerment. During a presentation at the African Regional Workshop on the Integrated Project, a participant noted:

> After ICPD [the Cairo Conference] we look at the issue of larger human development and gender. In the next ten years we will be changing from "national family planning program" to "reproductive health program" or "gender and development" program.[41]

The official presentations at the conference emphasized the move to embrace broader issues of women's reproductive health and their link to women's empowerment. The Congratulatory Address given by the executive director of the project's donor agency exemplifies this rhetorical commitment:

> These global conferences have placed human beings at the centre of population and development activities, bringing our attention to the needs for comprehensive reproductive health care including family planning, and empowerment of women (Kon 1995).

However, my fieldwork suggest that the project pushed women to become empowered to make decisions against childbearing at home, but not to make decisions of a political nature including distribution of project spoils or setting of project priorities. The Integrated Project could potentially contribute to women's empowerment in different ways. First, its scope could broadly extend into health and welfare issues. A project document states that: "family planning is basically a welfare matter and therefore it should be linked more closely with family health and welfare than with population control alone" (Tanzania Food and Nutrition Centre 1995, 52). The Integrated Project also addresses feminist goals because it is community based rather than centered within the medical establishment. Helzner and Shepard (1997) suggest that the CBD approach, which has local villagers, mostly women, as service providers, "fits better with a feminist ideal." They note that "this model significantly increases the chances that a woman's choice of family planning method will be voluntary because the relationship between her and the provider is more likely to be characterized by equality and respect" (1997, 177). However, they were less sanguine about other feminist concerns, such as the quality of information and service given by people with limited medical knowledge. In the project, women's empowerment was still the means for increasing family planning and decreasing fertility, not an end in itself.

The project also promotes feminist goals by encouraging women-specific development activities at the grassroots (Rowlands 1998). Material benefits from income-generating projects could meet women's strategic needs. Also, as Wieringa (1994), argues, "any project concerned with women can potentially entail a transformative element" so some income-generating projects may address women's strategic gender needs as well. In sum, the integrated project had the potential to contribute to women's empowerment but the shift to demographic and development goals undermined this potential.

But, negotiating the space between local priorities for men as well as women to benefit from women's development projects and funders' desire to increase family planning has depoliticized gender issues. The project assumes that since most participants are women, they necessarily benefit from the project. However, the competing demands of donors and local communities converge during project implementation in ways that reinforce existing local gender inequalities and effectively allow men to usurp most of the potential benefits of the project.

One of the strategies for achieving feminist goals recommended by project documentation was "empowerment of the community particularly women in decision making" (Urrio 1995, 28). While women's empowerment was an official project goal, the perception that UMATI was focusing unduly on women threatened to exacerbate local-level gender conflicts. For example, UMATI held a weeklong seminar for training traditional birth attendants from 15 of the surrounding villages. Local men sitting outside the seminar were heard to complain in the quote introducing this section: women were working the international development system to their benefit and their male neighbors were displeased about it.

The idea that women, who are "just farmers," would receive project spoils, while men are left out, challenged local gender relations. Not only were these beneficiaries women, but were "just farmers" implying that they held no political clout. Projects rarely succeed without support from locally powerful figures—generally men. To succeed, the project had to give enough benefits to men to ensure cooperation and reduce jealousy. At the same time, UMATI tried to appear committed to the post-Cairo emphasis on women's empowerment.

Distributing benefits became even more difficult in the context of Tanzania's economic adjustment. A 1995 report recommended that "Local Steering Committee members and CBDs be used to sensitize the community on the need for them to share costs on the services they receive in this project" (UMATI 1995b, 10). This trend toward cost sharing in the project reflects international donor's determination to decrease dependence on aid and increase community payment for development services. These pressures have reduced the project spoils available to participants, particularly women.

Initially all project CBDs were women, so to the extent that personal gain came from participation, women benefited. However, as the project expanded and the larger context changed, it came under increasing pressure to involve men in family planning. Men were brought in as CBDs in addition to those who had already been involved on the Steering Committee. This satisfied the most powerful and vocal members of the villages by offering them part of the spoils. However, the question remained—were these male participants actually going to be contraceptive users? If only contraceptive users could benefit directly from project activities, was this not coercing poor villagers to use family planning?

These issues converged in the creation of a new project beneficiary: the "passive acceptor." At the African Regional Workshop on the project, the notion of passive acceptors was seen as a way to increase the numbers of beneficiaries. Passive acceptors are people who supposedly supported, but did not necessarily use family planning. In one village, for example, there were 20 CBDs but many project-supported income-generating groups. Another village had "52 members who contribute [to an income-generating project] but only one CBD—the rest are converts of family planning." This village government gave four acres of land to males who were "believers" and who practice family planning.[42] It seems the village leaders wanted to make the point that males as well as females could be involved in the projects and be "family planners."

Many people associated with the project supported the inclusion of passive acceptors and the expansion of family planning to include programs on reproductive health.[43] For example, a priest in Bati who had opposed UMATI began telling his parishioners that UMATI projects were good for the community. A project official explained that income-earning projects now provided benefits for passive supporters as well as CBDs and family planning users.[44] He approved of this change, for otherwise the project could be seen as coercive. The creation of the category, passive acceptors, thus managed to expand male participation in the project without challenging male reluctance to use contraception.

The notion of passive acceptors has implications for the project's feminist and demographic agendas. If donors want to reduce population through contraception, how can they be sure which acceptors are real and which are passive? When seed money or project supplies are offered as incentives for participation in the project, does this necessarily translate into contraceptive use? Are the acceptors contraceptive users or just people willing to participate in a project that has family planning as one of it components? If men are legitimate beneficiaries, both as CBDs and passive acceptors, how can the project ensure that unequal gender relations do not translate into male dominance of the project?

The implications of the passive acceptor for feminist goals are that project participation is no longer reserved either exclusively or primarily for women. For example, at CBD and Local Steering Committee meetings, men dominated conversation and continually pushed their own agendas to the forefront. Including men in women's groups may, in theory, expose them to more progressive ideas on women's health issues and women's empowerment. However, in practice, with no structural means of diffusing existing gender biases, men are able to use these inequalities to expand their own control within the project.

Conclusions

This chapter has demonstrated how development, demographic, and feminist narratives underlie the implementation of an integrated family planning project in Tanzania. The project has operated in a historically specific context that has affected its relationship to the state and its policies and practices. UMATI has had to compete with other organizations and prove the success of its interventions. While the project has been influenced by the Cairo discourse on women's reproductive health, with its feminist and development agendas, the structural adjustment programs and donor emphasis on demographic goals have taken precedence in actual implementation.

A development agenda, understood as responsiveness to local communities, usually perpetuates gendered biases in those communities. A demographic agenda of fertility reduction leads to a narrow focus on the family planning component of the project. When these two agendas compete with feminist goals to improve women's health and increase women's empowerment, the feminist goals are often ignored. At the local level, women are project beneficiaries in traditionally female spheres: by using the contraceptives provided to control their own fertility and by providing most of the labor for the project's activities. In contrast, men receive a disproportionate amount of the spoils from income-generating activities and control over the Local Steering Committees.

The important negotiating mechanism of category formation (Tilly 1999), understood by the new classification of the passive acceptor, demonstrates how effectively local actors can take new demands, like the feminist agenda of Cairo, and shape them using new and local categories. Rural women, supposedly the primary beneficiaries of the project, provide its justification—after all, it is their "problem" of profligate fertility that family planning is meant to "solve." They do most of the work—going door to door to provide contraception. While a voluntary project suggests a higher level of community responsiveness and involvement, it requires free time. Rural Tanzanian women are the most overworked members of their communities, and in periods of economic hardship, they have even less time to volunteer. Finally, they are blamed for failure since they are both the primary implementers and users of contraceptives.

Another important mechanism for power mediation is that of improvisation. As Tilly argues, "improvisation matters because it always takes place within limits set by existing social relations and locally shared understandings, then modifies existing social relations and locally shared understandings" (1999, 350). If local population projects such as the integrated project are to empower women, improvisation is perhaps the best term we can give to the kinds of actions necessary to do so. Yet, what interests could be expected to push for such initiatives—keeping in mind that such empowerment might spark resistance to the disempowering aspects of demographic and development agendas? The Local Steering Committee is hardly going to risk their role in the village community. "Local" NGOs, like UMATI, which depend on donor funding, are constrained by donor requirements. Other women's groups could mobilize at the grassroots for more project accountability on empowerment issues, but they would need an independent resource base. Furthermore, these groups would have to believe that an integrated approach to family planning and gender empowerment was worth the investment of their limited time and money. Finally, should we expect resistance from local women who are meant to benefit from the project, but are vulnerable both within the project and outside of it?

Because the integrated project has been situated in a historical framework that has favored integrating family planning with goals of women's empowerment and local-level community development, this project could demonstrate the possibilities for implementing the Cairo ideals, particularly the fit between feminist goals and the other project activities. Instead, it illustrates the need to give feminist goals explicit priority by international donors. If success at the national level is to be equated with increased contraceptive use by women, then the Cairo discourse becomes merely an auxiliary agenda. Therefore, until women's empowerment is seen as more than simply a means to decreased fertility levels, family planning projects may theoretically support a feminist agenda, but this will have little meaning in practice.

Intermezzo 2

Development in Theater and Practice: The Regional Workshop on the Integrated Project

The particular opportunities accorded to integrated projects provided the impetus for bringing together representatives from implementing countries to share their experiences in biannual conferences. With the permission of the MOH and the project's international donors during the first phase of my field research, I was an observer at the Regional Workshop on the Integrated Project from December 5–11, 1995. The workshop took place in a large conference room at the Kilimanjaro Hotel which, at that time, was the most exclusive hotel in Dar es Salaam. Delegates from African countries with existing or planned projects met to discuss ways to promote the integrated projects.[1] Also in attendance were representatives from UNFPA, IPPF, WHO, Pathfinder International, JOICFP, and the National Sales Manager for Smithcline Beecham in Nigeria.[2] Delegates sat arranged around a rectangular configuration of tables, with a podium and seats for distinguished guests at the front. The decorative and theatrical atmosphere suggested that I was about to view a performance, rather than a series of project workshops.[3]

The way in which "development" was performed said little about the actual integrated project itself, and even less about its participants; however, it did speak to the ways in which development projects are expected to work and to local people's ability to understand these expectations and perform their roles accordingly. The highlight of the conference came from a field trip to visit the project sites in Morogoro Region. This field trip epitomizes what Chambers (1983) terms "rural development tourism." The participants were typical rural development tourists whom Chambers aptly describes as:

> Differing widely in race, nationality, religion, profession, age, sex, language, interests, prejudices, conditioning and experience, these visitors nevertheless usually have three things in common: they come from urban areas; they want to find something out; and they are short of time (Chambers 1983, 11).

Indeed, most participants were high-level officials from various African health ministries or NGOs who had come from Dar es Salaam or their own capital cities. They were spending an entire day of their workshop in order to understand what was "really" happening in the project. Also, due to a late start, the location of the site, and the fact that everyone had to return to the hotel in the capital city for the night, participants were extremely short of time.

Participants left the Kilimanjaro Hotel in two mini-buses headed first for the more established Bati project (about 230 kilometers from Dar es Salaam and 1,400 meters in altitude in the Uluguru mountains) and then for the Mali project in the valley. The drive from Dar es Salaam to Morogoro town took approximately two and a half hours on a tarmac road, but the drive to Bati consisted of another two and a half hours on a dirt and rock road that wound its way up the mountain. The steep inclines and hairpin curves were quite unsettling to the conference participants, many of whom stated explicitly that they saw no reason why we actually had to take a field trip to see a project site. When the buses reached the entrance of Upana village, the commercial center of Bati Division, we were met by groups of local people. Women wearing their finest clothing or their CBD uniforms waved branches and sang while running alongside the two buses. When the buses arrived at the local government office square, project participants filed out amidst crowds of villagers singing, children dancing, and young men drumming on oil cans and playing other homemade instruments—all in celebration of the visitors. There was no sign from the local people that the project visitors had arrived over four hours later than planned, and the visitors did their part of dutifully signing the guest book and trying to appear interested, despite their weariness from the trip. The local dignitaries and project participants quickly organized themselves to get on with the show. Indeed, the visit was more ceremony than fact-finding mission.

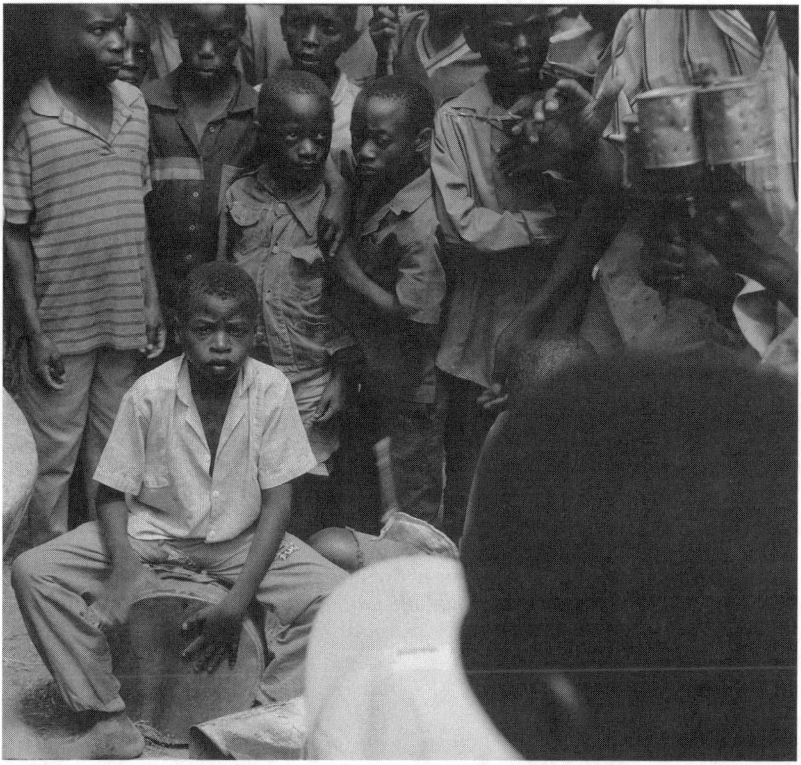

Photo 2 Young Boys Play Music to Entertain the Foreign Visitors in their IP Village
Source: Photograph by Lisa Ann Richey.

After a few minutes of song, the crowds were pushed to the periphery so that the central business between the IP visitors and their local development experts could begin. All TBA and CBD agents were dressed in their uniforms, some wearing badges with the National Family Planning Programme "green star" family planning logo. They sat together as a group on the edge of the concrete foundation, while the central figures, including all the visitors, were arranged on benches and chairs. A handful of local "big men" gave speeches, including one man in a Kaunda suit who had come up for the occasion from the district offices in town. Some speeches were given in English, a clear indicator of the education level of the speaker, while others were in Kiswahili and translated by the UMATI coordinator who led the

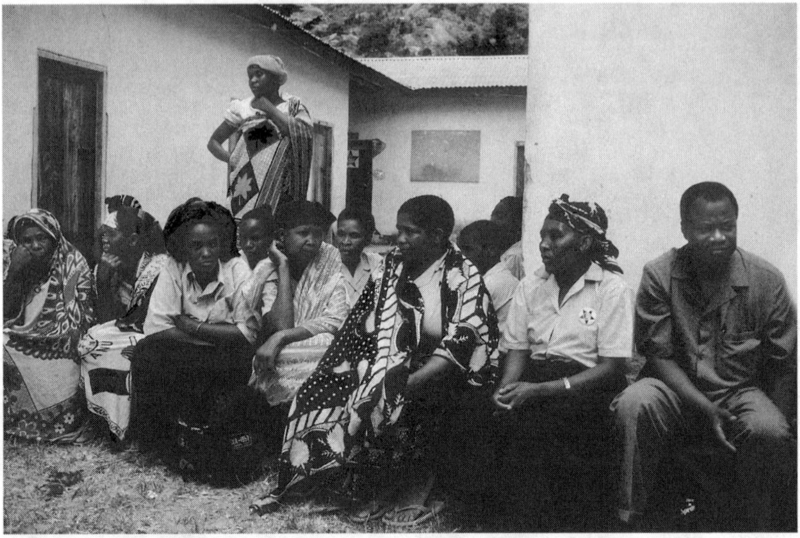

Photo 3 Traditional Birth Attendants, Community-Based Distributors of Family Planning, and a Local Government Official Watch the IP Ceremonies in their Village

Source: Photograph by Lisa Ann Richey.

group. The content of the speeches involved a summary of all the project activities in the village and their "successes." Family planning was quite conspicuous in its absence, with the emphasis given to income-generating projects. Every speech included the requisite words of appreciation to UMATI and to JOICFP for their support. The most "local" of the speakers was the project coordinator for Bati and Mali, who had been living at the Bati site. He listed directly the inputs given by JOICFP as: "building supplies, money, materials for CBDs such as bicycles, shoes, bags, uniforms and medicines."[4] The speeches were very formal and there was no time for discussion, as the agenda included a walking tour to see firsthand the various aspects of the project and time was at a premium. By this time, the local people who were not directly related to the presentation had dispersed, but the CBDs and TBAs continued along with the project visitors to "demonstrate" their activities.

After the long drive, followed by sitting in the afternoon sun, the visitors were quite tired and struggled to follow their hosts along the mountainous terrain from one site to another. Woven mats and earthen pots made by the CBDs and TBAs were offered for sale in one of the government offices. Sewing machines, donated by UMATI, were displayed in a shop alongside a few dresses and school uniforms as representative of the sewing project. Visitors were taken to see the stalls of two large pigs, part of the piggery project and then finally to the nursery school building where a toilet slab, piece of rudimentary laboratory equipment, and wilted pine saplings were displayed to represent the nursery school, toilet, deworming, and afforestation projects respectively.

The CBDs and TBAs politely posed for pictures, and, as in the archetype characterized by Chambers (1983), nervously responded to a few questions in ways which they hoped would bring benefits and avoid penalties. For example, one project visitor asked about how they actually sold the pine saplings that were located next to the nursery school, a considerable hike up from the center of the village. A CBD responded clearly that they sell them to whoever comes and asks for them. A number of visitors noted in English amongst themselves that these were problems of marketing and suggested that the potential marketability should be considered before these income-generating projects were started.

Having spent approximately two hours in total in Bati, the group coordinator apologized to the local people, and insisted that we had to leave to visit the site in Mali before returning to Dar es Salaam in the evening. The local people sang, danced, and drummed as we all boarded the buses, perhaps in a gratitude that we had come, or perhaps because we were leaving and the village could be returned to normal.

The visit to Mali was quite similar to that in Bati, with singing and dancing welcoming the distinguished visitors.[5] However, due to time constraint, speeches and tours were cut down significantly, and the visitors became outspoken about their own tiredness. The walking portion of the tour was substituted by a drive over to one of the sites for baking bricks, part of the "brick-making project" where, depending on who was explaining the project, bricks were either being made to use for building a future UMATI office, or for selling to benefit project participants. Some of the visitors suggested that they would prefer to stay in the bus, instead of looking at the brick making in progress, but the group coordinator insisted that such behavior would hurt the feelings of the Mali contingent who were very proud of their project and wanted to show it off.

When the end of the tour seemed imminent, one influential visitor from the project's funder, JOICFP, asked to see the local clinic that provided backup services for family planning. This had not been part of the planned agenda, but as the clinic was on the road heading back to town, and a donor representative was requesting it, both vans made an unanticipated visit to the local clinic. By this time it was early evening, so the clinic was officially closed. However, since the medical assistant in-charge lived in the back rooms of the clinic, he cordially welcomed the visitors, and brought out the clinic guest book to be passed around while visitors milled about, examined the family planning posters, and asked a few polite questions about the clinic. At the end of the day, all of the exhausted visitors boarded their mini-buses to return to the Kilimanjaro Hotel in the capital, perhaps with the notion that they had seen the "real" integrated project of the "remote" villages in Morogoro Region.

On the following day of the conference, participants were invited to ask questions in response to the field trip that were then answered by the area service delivery manager who had been the tour leader. One participant expressed disappointment that we were not able to see the family planning component, so we were unclear on how the family planning program was progressing in the project sites. He went on to suggest that he thought that we might have been able to visit the home of an "acceptor" to talk to her about family planning.[6] The participant was informed that the conference theme was "sustainability of CBD," so we looked particularly at those aspects of the project and not at others.

The PANFRICO V workshop illustrates many of the expectations that donors and implementing agencies have of the project. As the Tanzanian host, UMATI was expected to perform the role of effective project implementer. In order to do this, speeches had to be well written to document the successes of the project in all areas, but most importantly, local people in the project villages visited had to perform appropriately. The various project components were expected to be well-integrated, so that participation in projects designed to address community needs would build solidarity between men and women in the villages, and between local people and UMATI. The anticipated outcome of this development effort is increased family planning use, as men and women are sensitized and become more comfortable with the issue and as the resources are made available locally through CBD agents supplied by UMATI. Local people are, of course, expected to be gracious and enthusiastic, showing that they are indeed in need of donor assistance, but also willing to "help themselves."

At the same time, the ambivalences and conflicting agenda inherent within the project itself emerged repeatedly during the workshop. How can the project respond to local needs by focusing on poverty alleviation and income generation, when it is "in the business of family planning"? How can the project draw in local support on the basis of its identity as a development project, when family planning is not among the priorities of local communities? How can the project simultaneously build up "the community at the grassroots" and focus on "weaning the project sites for eventual self-sustainability"? Negotiating the contrasted and competing agenda is a formidable task for UMATI, which must bridge fundamentally different expectations from radically different constituencies.

5

Identities, Expectations, and Control: Negotiating Traditional Practices and Modern Methods

Introduction: "Tradition," "Modernity," and Hegemonies

Population policies are state interventions into some of the most intimate and private aspects of citizens' lives. Both the benefits of family planning for those who desire it, and the possibilities of coercion against those who do not, are well-known aspects of international population policies. As described in chapter three, such policies are implemented through donor-funded family planning programs that promote modern contraceptives (see Warwick 1982). This development intervention (Ferguson 1994) arises out of the view, known as the demographic paradigm (Freedman 1999), that overpopulation is a fundamental development obstacle. Population control, a manifestation of self-discipline or governmentality, is linked to the larger neoliberal project of development. Because a considerable part of the "othering" of Africans involves a disproportionate interest in their sexuality (Mohanty 1991), control over reproduction holds particular weight in signifying an ability to control one's self.

This chapter uses data collected in clinics in Morogoro, Kilimanjaro, and Ruvuma Regions of Tanzania to understand how notions of modernity in the family planning program construct female bodies as "traditional" and "modern," how these discursive inequalities reflect and compound material disparities and how these logics come into play in the ways that women construct themselves and each other. As such, it analyzes both how population knowledge is distributed and how it is evaluated along the way. As described in chapter one, discipline is rational, impersonal, and neutral, yet the political implications of how discipline is wielded run along recognizable cleavages of race, class, and gender. Family planning technologies, more than simply a means for preventing conception, are involved as identity artifacts in the construction of bodies and in the reproduction of power relations. As such, modern contraceptives, organized by and implemented through donor-funded programs constitute a discursive apparatus through which scattered hegemonies are disseminated.

The term "scattered hegemonies" is useful in describing the character of relationships of power that are simultaneously both hegemonic and plural (Grewal and Kaplan 1994). These scattered hegemonies come out of the globalization of ideas, mobile capital, and multiple subjectivities. Acting in conjunction with other patriarchal discourses of controlling women's bodies, the hegemony of the definition of population as a problem and modern family planning as its solution becomes scattered throughout all levels of the Tanzanian experience. The global population discourse, service providers' constructions of identity, expectations of local communities, and control of husbands, are all sites for both compliance and resistance. Women's use of family planning, traditional and modern, allows them to counter the expectations of these hegemonies at some times, and to embody them at others.

In order to transmit modern family planning as the mechanism for regulating diverse bodies and populations, the population discourse implicitly constructs a particular African body, essentially the same, and essentially different from its referent, the white, middle-class Western woman (Oudshoorn 1996). When this laboratory body and real bodies and practices do not match, negotiation and definition takes place at the local level. Service providers have their own vested interests in the opportunity to increase their own symbolic and material capital in a context of economic struggle. However, they must negotiate the fit between the expectations from above that bodies are the same, and the realities from below that bodies are different. The bodies in question are indexing Tanzanian women (Bordo 1990) who find themselves at the centre of a complex web of power relations in which there is no level playing field for the negotiation of health services (see Whiteford and Manderson 2000).

As chapters two and three describe, international donors and lenders have shaped national population policy and family planning interventions. This chapter demonstrates how clinic-level contraception has been shaped by the priorities of Tanzania's donors and lenders, as well as by the crisis in state social service provision as I describe in detail elsewhere (Richey 2004). The Tanzanian program followed the discursive shift from population control to improving reproductive health after the 1994 Cairo Conference, with the re-named National Reproductive and Child Health Programme. However, such a diverse and expensive agenda has proven difficult to implement. In practice, vestiges of global population control ideology are laid over local prejudices to form new modes of identity distinction and control. I am not arguing here that modern contraceptives should not be made available to Third World women, simply that their prioritization in the Tanzanian family planning program reflects an interest in contraceptive continuity, not one in increasing the choice of individual women. As Bledsoe, Banja, and Hill (1998) argue from their case study in the Gambia, most African women are not only happy to have contraceptive options; they would probably like more. Farmer (1999) convincingly argues that critical scholars need to avoid the "Luddite trap" where addressing the social roots of disease is held to be incompatible with advocating the delivery of high-quality, high-tech healthcare. However, technology, as we all know, is never neutral; thus feminist critiques of technology and policy can provide useful tools for analyzing contraceptive meanings.[1] In the context of international population policy, this needs to be read alongside work linking feminist theory with class, race, and technoscience (see for example, Clarke and Olesen 1999) to provide a critical perspective for examining population policies whose targets are primarily poor, black women.

In the next section, I examine how notions of tradition and modernity are defined at different policy levels. Section three investigates the ways the service providers themselves embody the apparatus of family planning. Then section four describes family planning's identity artifacts and examines the constructions of identity that take place between service providers and their clients. In section five, I examine some of the practices of reproductive control that Tanzanian women use to acknowledge, respond to, and challenge these different powers over their bodies. In the final section, I draw some conclusions about how popular dichotomies between traditional/modern, compliance/resistance and essential/constructed become unintelligible in the context of the lives of Tanzanian women.

Making Contraceptive Methods Traditional and Modern

Contraceptives take meaning from the contexts in which they are understood: they are both technological facts and mental conceptions (Russell and Thompson 2000, 4). The term modern is used to describe behavioral patterns and fertility desires that bring about a "demographic transition" (see Kirk 1996) as well as the types of contraceptive technologies that should assist couples in realizing these goals. In Tanzania these have been: pills, IUD, injection [Depo-Provera], diaphragm/foam/jelly, condom, female sterilization and male sterilization (Ngallaba et al. 1991/1992, 31). Implementing national population policies in Africa rests primarily on the provision of modern contraceptives for limiting and spacing births. Yet, communities in Tanzania also have various traditional ways for achieving these ends.

One way that service providers construct their own identities within the clinic setting is to contrast them to identities and practices known as traditional. However, this identification is not merely local in its genesis. There is both an international and a national context of discourses on tradition in terms of family planning. Contraceptive practices, in their use and discussion, can become signs for larger conceptualizations of the modern or lack of it (see Rutenberg and Watkins 1997 for similar evidence from Kenya). While using modern family planning is certainly not the only way of signifying one's modernity, it provides the opportunity for asserting an identity that is progressive, regulated, scientific, and Western. This identity is embedded in the international population discourse and passed down to service providers and local women through the apparatus of modern family planning.[2]

Within the international population discourse, traditional contraception is, at best, a poor choice of means for achieving the goal of fertility control. As Johnson-Hanks elaborates, "some program-oriented groups do not consider 'traditional' methods to be contraception at all" (2002, 229). Methods labeled traditional in the Tanzanian Demographic and Health Survey (DHS) have been limited to three types: "periodic abstinence (rhythm method), mucus method, and withdrawal" (Ngallaba 1991/1992, 31), or by the 1999 survey "mucus method" had been replaced with "lactational amenorrhoea." Most of the methods described by women in interviews as traditional contraceptives fall outside of the DHS categories of tradition. The traditional methods that count for the official discourse are those that modern science documents as being somewhat effective, and thus, tradition is redefined according to the progress of modern science. A telling example from a neighboring country, Uganda, illustrates this point. In the Ugandan DHS, the categories were redefined to classify breastfeeding as a modern contraceptive. It was explained to me at the official dissemination of the survey that science had now confirmed breastfeeding as an effective method. Thus, breastfeeding has been redefined as modern, while tradition is a category reserved for methods whose effectiveness remains scientifically unverified.

Any method of family planning usage, however effective, may also be understood as a sign of the desire to prevent conception and the power, to some degree, to do so. The Senior Population Program Specialist in one of the donor missions told me "withdrawal is an unusually common method in Tanzania." He went on to say that "there are some people who don't trust modern methods." When I asked about the religious-based service providers who are teaching "natural" family planning he said, "if someone has five kids and is using natural contraception then they are just stupid!" Of course, taking into consideration that the average desired fertility at the time was approximately six children, it would seem that couples in the scenario described by the specialist might have been successfully achieving their fertility objectives. Nonetheless, they were not successful modern family planners.

Traditional methods are conspicuous in their absence in donor documents, minutes, and publications. However, one exception is the discussion of how traditional family planning methods reflect a larger problem for international family planning promoters—the traditional mindset that serves as a barrier to the adoption of contraceptives. An entire section on "Traditional Values, Beliefs and Attitudes" of a paper entitled "The Social Soundness of Supporting Family Planning in Tanzania" explains the traditions that "contribute to, and support high fertility."[3] This list contains an eclectic mix of beliefs and practices, some relating to material conditions or practices, and others to attitudes, that perpetuate what Uma Narayan has called "blaming culture" (Narayan 1997). "Bad culture" is to be countered programmatically by educational messages promoting the small family norm. Typical of modernization discourses, tradition is characterized by a lack of knowledge and the assumption that if people just knew better, they would abandon their traditional ideas.

At the national level, traditional and modern descriptively reflect the dual contexts in which Tanzanians at this level find themselves as described in detail in chapter three—implementing a population policy that is funded by donors and situated firmly within the global population discourse, and at the same time, aware that many family planning practices existed both before the introduction of modern family planning and outside its scope. Tanzanians responsible for implementing the population policy construct their own category of traditional contraceptives with their correlating users, traditional women. These methods take on a mythical historical meaning, emphasizing that in the past, Tanzanians were capable of controlling their own fertility and they had the means to do so. Therefore there is a thread that links modern family planning's biomedical contraceptives with Tanzanian tradition (see also Watkins 2000 on Kenya).

The notion that traditional family planning was lost knowledge was explained, to my surprise, by a senior statistician in the Planning Commission working on the population policy. He told me that he was interested in knowing more about traditional family planning methods:

> How did they work? Perhaps there are different conditions now, but we need to find out more about them. People won't reveal the traditional methods...for example, my mother had only 3 children. How did she do it?[4]

Other informants also told me that the generation of their parents (or grandparents) knew how to space children. This knowledge had somehow been lost in the transitions between generations, so "now people don't know how to space and they are getting pregnant every year."[5]

The portrayal of traditional methods as lost knowledge is interesting for two reasons. First, it implies that both the motivation and the means for childspacing were in existence before the introduction of modern family planning services. Thus, childspacing is not a foreign import, but an offshoot from indigenous knowledge. As described in chapter two, this has important political implications for policymakers and implementers who want to stress the ways in which the population policy is a *Tanzanian* response to *Tanzanian* needs as opposed to being an imposition by outsiders. This knowledge has somehow been lost (or corrupted, or eclipsed) by the new regime of modern family planning. Responses to this transition are either that more research needs to be done to reclaim this lost knowledge, or that couples should now adopt modern methods that are of the same nature as methods used traditionally in the past.

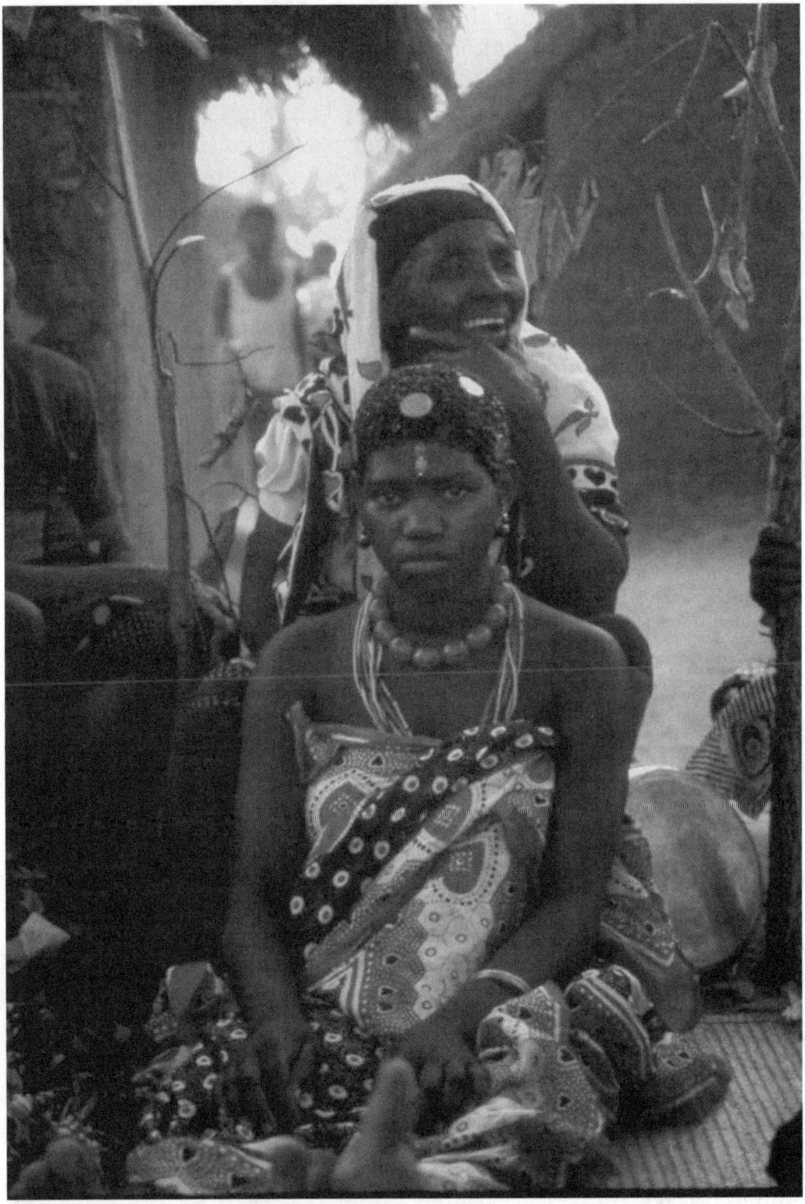

Photo 4 A Young Yao Woman is Celebrating Her *unyago* Initiation Ceremony, Now Held after the Birth of Her First Child

Source: Photograph by Lisa Ann Richey.

A second issue that stands out from the conceptualization of traditional methods as lost knowledge is that these methods are being equated with their modern equivalents. Therefore, instead of considering traditional family planning as a behavioral process (such as postpartum abstinence, withdrawal, or prolonged breastfeeding) it is considered, like modern methods, as a *device* that one uses to prevent births.[6] Therefore, when the knowledge of what this thing was or how it was used is lost, it is no longer functional as a family planning method. When the traditional devices are no longer a viable option, modern methods offer a convenient and effective substitute. The effectiveness of the behavioral methods of family planning relied on involvement of both sexual partners, while, except for the condom, the modern devices' reliability and effectiveness are dependent on female efficacy.

This shift from old bodies to new ones was explained as inevitable with the changing times. For example, when I asked CBD agents of a family planning village project about traditional methods they described the following method of *kuweka pigi* [a method involving tying a string around your waist to prevent conception]:

> In the past these worked well but today the *waganga* [traditional healers] are not like the *waganga* in the past. People have no faith—they can't use them today, so today we have *njia za kisasa* [modern contraceptives]. These traditional methods have expired.[7]

Even after skeptical probing, the CBDs all agreed that the traditional methods had worked well in the past. I was surprised to find service providers explaining the effectiveness of a traditional method. Most service providers, as I will explore later, exclusively associate themselves with the provision and use of modern methods. However, these providers all agreed that the *pigi*, a popular method with some of my respondents, was considered a legitimate method—in the past. By adding the time dimension, they could maintain their own modern identity, as the distributors of *njia za kisasa* [modern contraceptives] while also recognizing that many people did (and do) use traditional methods. Echoing the discourse of policymakers, there is a construction of a loss of knowledge due to the failure of contemporary traditional healers coupled with the loss of faith of their clients.

A central link between family planning and modern women's body identity came out during an informal conversation with a service provider who had been working at a regional hospital in maternal and child health for many years. She explained that times have changed and women do not want as many children as their parents had: "You see women who have had many children—they have breasts that hang down to here [she demonstrated with her hands cupped at her stomach]—breasts like socks!"

This description of how non-modern women embody their backwardness in "breasts like socks" holds an implicit comparison to a universal modern ideal woman who would never have so many children as to compromise her body's aesthetic qualities (or at least she would not have to breastfeed them all). The interpretation by the service provider of this woman's exaggerated fecundity as embodied in her breasts is a physical manifestation of the link between femininity, maternity, and excess. Such breasts might have represented many different things: maternal generosity, physical depletion, or simply normal aging. I think this also suggests that the situatedness of the service provider between the international population discourse and the local-level women over whom she is to be an authority shapes the ways in which women read notions of tradition and modernity into bodies. The service provider is creating the sense the inappropriate conditions exist for the next pregnancy, thus in a very nuanced way, interpreting the global population discourse in relevant local demographies as the next chapter elaborates.

Service Providers Embody Modern Family Planning

In local clinics, modern family planning has come to signify a transition to modern bodies constructed simultaneously vis-à-vis their non-modern sisters. The ways that modern bodies are constructed as identities has both local and global dimensions. Service providers signify their modernity by learning the lessons of their training in "Comprehensive Family Planning," passing this knowledge on to others, and also by embodying this very knowledge.

A district-level MCH coordinator elaborated on the reasons women now think of children in terms of resources spent per child:

> In the past two or three years, life has gotten much more difficult—now you have to pay for everything for children. Also because of cost-sharing—people have gotten the idea to reduce their family size. Even extended families have begun to change. Workers used to have 4 or 5

> children, but now they are thinking of 2 or 3 at most. It is different than in years past. If you have to advise others to space and limit their children, then you have to set an example. Now, especially family planning service providers have changed a lot and they use family planning often.[8]

I was surprised that when I asked her questions meant to elicit her professional viewpoint about how family planning clients were reacting to socioeconomic change, she responded to me from a personal level. Perhaps not about her own life per se, but about the lives of women, such as herself: workers and family planning service providers. These women were the ones who really understood the changes going on around them. They had the insight to recognize the instability brought about by economic restructuring and, as they had been taught at during seminars, sensitization workshops, and technical training sessions, had adjusted their behavior appropriately. They had taken on new modern bodies and identities in response to the demands of the realities of modern economic life.

The importance of modern family planning offers interesting opportunities for some Tanzanian women who serve as "go-betweens" brokering these imported technologies. In ways that parallel the negotiations described in chapter two between the Tanzanian state and its donors and lenders, service providers are able to use the population discourse strategically to build their own symbolic and economic capital (see Bourdieu 1991). The more important the problem of population in official terms, the more significant the role of those persons responsible for solving the problem. This status is deepened by donor commitment to funding the national program. At the same time, family planning as the preeminent solution to women and children's health problems provides legitimacy from below. Infant and child mortality and morbidity, maternal mortality, poor nutrition, and disease are all locally felt health needs. Therefore, interventions that purport to deal with these important problems are welcomed. Local level service providers are equipped with the tools that can enable women to control their fertility, and serve their families and nation through limited childbearing. One of the standard health education [*elimu ya afya*] talks, entitled "The benefits of using family planning" included a demographic explanation by the service provider: "If there are less people, the government can provide better services, and there will be more children with education." The benefit to the nation as a whole if individual women will use family planning attempts to link personal incentives with demographic considerations: harnessing the energies of the individual toward regulation of the population.

Situating Knowledge, Identity Artifacts, and Negotiating Bodies

> *We don't like to intrude [kuingia sana] but if Mama has too much work she can always forget to take pills, or if Baba is a drunkard, then Mama will have difficulties with family planning.*[9]

The ideology and identity artifacts of modern family planning reproduce power relations of the international population discourse to be interpreted in the local context. Service providers are, almost always, Tanzanian women, but family planning as a series of practices embedded in global relations of competing and unequally funded development agenda provides a means by which service providers can distinguish themselves from their clients. Family planning service providers are marked or identified at the clinic level by their knowledge of modern methods. These technologies are designed for bodies that are the same, but when they are implemented in the real world context, bodies are different. Service providers are then in the difficult position of negotiating between the needs of the different bodies and the expectations of the family planning apparatus.

Family planning service provision as an impetus for donor funding has provided a channel for personal and professional gain. Contrary to my expectations before going to the field that family planning may be resisted in vociferously Catholic areas or that the increased repertoire of services and demands on an overtaxed health care system would be resented, all service providers expressed positive dispositions toward the provision of modern family planning. Service providers want to become trained in family planning because training means attending classes, usually in the regional capital city, where they are given room, board, and a per diem. Completion of this training also opens up avenues for future training—refresher courses, specialized courses, or expansion of basic training all provide another opportunity for increased material and symbolic capital. These professional opportunities are particularly welcomed in the context of scarcity resulting from the history of economic crisis (see Raikes 1992).

The power of language came up in my research as one important theme characterizing the relationship between service providers and clients.[10] Poststructuralist and critical theory have drawn attention to the need to recognize language as more than simply a choice of words, but as a channel for other forms of power (Bourdieu 1991, Foucault 1979). The analysis of language used, as well as things unsaid, can provide grounds for interpreting meaning within a given context. Language is important for signifying authority, drawing boundaries, and creating communities. English instead of Kiswahili is the family planning language in areas of training, educational materials, and supervision. I conducted all of my research in Kiswahili, and initially I considered the idea that perhaps service providers were using English words in my presence in an attempt to help me understand what they were doing. However, as time passed and I saw the same juxtaposition of English with Kiswahili, even in written materials that were obviously not meant particularly for my observation, I began to understand the use of English as a signifier of one's expertise, professionalism, and ultimately one's modernity.

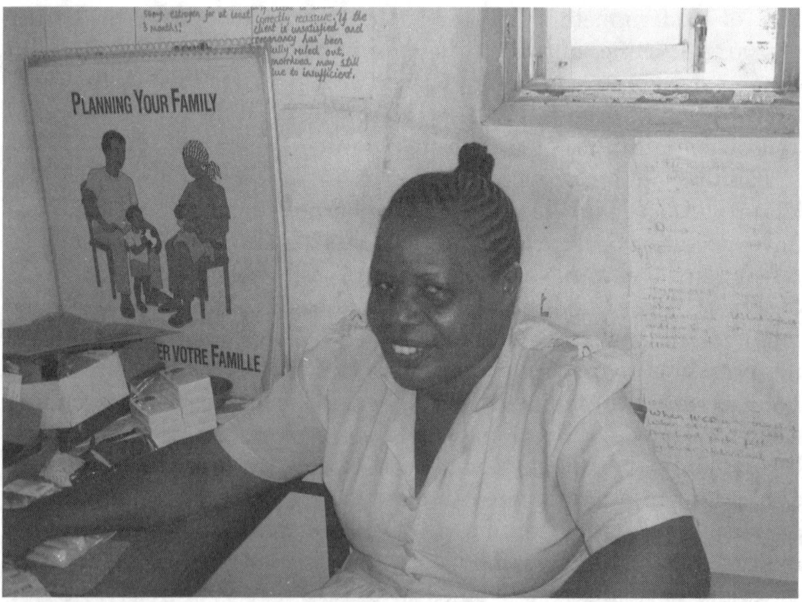

Photo 5 A Trained Family Planning Service Provider at Her Desk in a Regional Hospital

Source: Photograph by Lisa Ann Richey.

The presence of English as the family planning language can be attributed at one level to imported knowledge about imported technologies—the contraceptives themselves are manufactured in English-speaking places, the technical advisors who come to support the Ministry of Health are English speaking, and the overseas training and study tours given by donors to top-level officials take place in English-speaking environments. However, at another level, the choice to use English in a context where the majority of those hearing it would not understand its meaning acts as a signifier of service providers' access to specialized knowledge and control over its corresponding technologies.

Training of service providers occurs through rote memorization of precepts in English with little attempt to situate them in a social/cultural context. However, it does situate providers as educated women of high status. Service providers inviting me to observe when counseling was being conducted for new clients said things like, "*Twende. Sasa tunafanya* informed choice" [Let's go. Now we are going to do "informed choice"]. The English words inserted in Kiswahili discussions had meaning only to me, other highly educated listeners, and service providers trained in family planning. Very few clients would have any idea what was about to be done to them. Also, during training, service providers made educational posters depicting intervention flow charts, potentially dangerous side effects associated with specific family planning methods, and even clients' rights in English. These posters were then brought back to the service provider's clinic and displayed on the walls. However, aside from telling foreign visitors that family planning was taking place at the clinic, these materials did little to improve the quality of care at the clinics because most were incomprehensible to the majority of their viewers. Few, if any, of the clients could read the posters stating their rights in family planning clinics. Few, if any, service providers read them after the training seminars were over, and they often had difficulty explaining what the message meant in practice. The unintended result of the production of educational materials in English is to remind clients of the gaps between themselves and the service providers who are supposedly able to understand the foreign messages. Finally, the family planning supervision guidelines were similarly done in English.[11] I observed family planning supervision in one district and witnessed first-hand the difficulties of supervision-in-translation. While in theory, anyone who would be responsible for supervision at this level would have been able to understand English, in practice, using guidelines that are written in

English demands that more time and energy be put into translation than in supervision itself. Questions involving more difficult concepts, often surrounding provider-client interaction and/or sensitive issues of reproductive health, were skipped over to save time. Most questions meant to assess quality of care issues were translated into Kiswahili with the equivalent of "Do you have any problems with [issue for evaluation]?" Not surprisingly, in a culture where stoic responses are the norm, there was almost no indication of any problems in the clinics. Priority was given to the meticulous collection of service provision statistics from the clinic records as required by the national program and its donors. While English served as a bridge between local family planning and international consultants and funders, it served as a barrier between providers and their clients.

Modern family planning comes to the clinic with its own set of tools and supplies. These things distinguish it from other less funded, and therefore, apparently less important, clinic activities. In light of the international discourse on quality of care that should be received by clients in family planning clinics, Tanzanian clinics are supposed to be brought up to standard for providing services. Most of this improvement is predicated on restructuring other clinic activities so that family planning will have its own room. Ideally, clients will be counseled and examined in rooms that guarantee their privacy. Donors fund limited improvements to clinics that will be used as training sites for family planning courses. At one such site where I worked, the MCH coordinator explained:

> When the clinic became a training site for family planning, they did renovations on the building, provided instruments, a lamp, bed, cabinet, sterilizer—all coming from the FPU [family planning unit]. At the time of training, the students come with soap, *jik* [bleach], and gloves.... We get higher morale for our work with family planning because we have gotten proper books for keeping records in, etc. (Participant observation fieldnotes, August 12, 1996).

As indicated by the MCH coordinator, the perception of higher morale due to a more professional environment is important. I would suggest that this is true even though the improvements brought into the clinic by its association with modern family planning are often only a coat of paint over crumbling walls. These things that come together with the family planning ideology act as identity artifacts: creating an identity for those women who control them.

Service providers are in the position of translating and interpreting these methods for their clients. However, the methods were designed with a preconfigured user whose body is not the same as the bodies in the Tanzanian context (see Oudshoorn 1996). Drawing on Kuhlmann and Babitsch's (2002) attempt to reconcile constructivist and materialist perspectives on the body and health through a reading of Haraway (1991) and Grosz (1994), a different context makes a different body. Nutrition, exposure to disease, physical activity levels, pregnancy and childbearing histories are all markedly different between one context and another. The assumption by the global population discourse is that Tanzanian bodies are the same in so far as they can be expected to resemble laboratory results and Western women's bodies regarding contraceptive effectiveness and side effects. However, they are ultimately defined as different bodies that do not need the same level of care as Western bodies, justifying culturally relative notions of quality.[12] Modern methods themselves come with a preconfigured body context that may or may not be present in Tanzania. Norplant insertions require a sterile surgical environment and a skilled technician trained in their insertion and removal. IUDs require a sexual relationship that does not expose the user to disease and regular internal examinations by a health care provider. Contraceptive pills must be stored in a dry place away from vermin and must be taken at regular intervals. All of these methods require that a woman not be pregnant when she begins them, with possible adverse effects to the developing fetus if she has already conceived. The connection between bodies, the body politic, and the political economy of development intertwine in ways that confront the reductionist notions of a technical fix to the population problem.

As I describe in more detail elsewhere (Richey 2003), Tanzanian clinics were lacking in expendable supplies such as gloves, necessary for examinations, bleach for sterilization of instruments, and sometimes syringes for injections. Service providers told women to buy their own expendables to bring to the clinic if they wanted a method that required them. Clean water supply, blood pressure cuffs, and pregnancy tests were regularly missing in all of the government clinics where I worked—even the regional hospitals. The existence of proper lighting is assumed in the implementation of many modern contraceptives and in any manifestation of the examination. During one day of clinic observation, service providers attempted to do a pelvic examination for an IUD insertion in a rural health center where there was no electricity, and no battery or solar-powered light.[13] They had a difficult time seeing well enough to conduct the exam and were faced with the dilemma of how to cope when the environment itself limited their ability to provide good quality of care. Opening the curtain would violate the client's right to privacy, as the examining room looked out onto the busy hospital courtyard; leaving it closed would leave the room in darkness. One service provider tried to manipulate the curtain to let in a thin stream of light while the other attempted to perform the examination. They had to direct the client to move down on the table to position her body in the ray of light so that they could examine her. Two service providers in turn looked into the woman's body. Unsure of their expertise in this situation, they asked me to help them, to which I politely declined, as I have no medical training. The client's own body presented an uncooperative circumstance. The young woman had come seeking contraception, but upon examination it was determined that she was already pregnant. After the exam, knowledge of this pregnancy was translated aloud by the service providers to the woman to indicate that she could not receive the IUD, and she should expect another baby. When the client had left, the service providers expressed their frustration to me, telling me how difficult it was to do their work in such an awkward context.

The overall disjuncture between modern technologies as identity artifacts and the material context in which these service providers are operating also contributes to a certain construction of women's practices and bodies as non-modern and therefore thwarting the correct usage of these technologies, and thus limits women's access to certain methods. Service providers regularly told me that women were forgetful, and thus could not be trusted to take a pill. Women were also commonly scolded by service providers when they came to the clinic without their appointment card, or if they came on any day, earlier or later than their prescribed return date (see also Allen 2004). Providers told me that they write the name of the client's 10-cell leader on their MCH card to ensure that in case they need to find a woman, they can track her down. These women themselves could not be trusted to discipline their bodies into the proper regime of childbearing and contraception.

While a "cafeteria approach" with a choice of methods is provided in theory, the items that are given preference in training of service providers and in presentation to clients are determined primarily by how effectively they promote the disciplining of women's bodies. As one service provider in a rural clinic on Mt. Kilimanjaro explained to me: "If you see a woman, you can look at her and you will know if she is likely to forget, and then you should advise her—'Why don't you use an IUD.'"

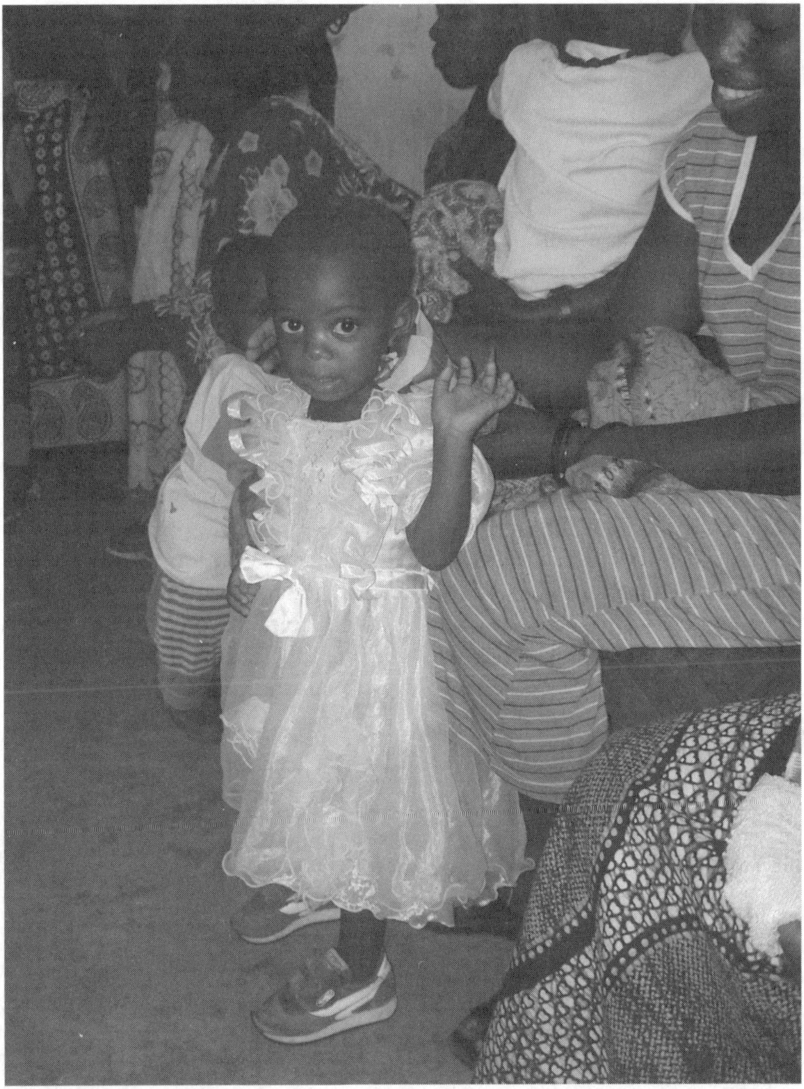

Photo 6 A Very Well-dressed Girl Accompanies Her Mother to an Urban Family Planning Clinic

Source: Photograph by Lisa Ann Richey.

Service providers are accustomed to "looking over" and "sizing up" their clients to access their contraceptive needs. How a client and her children are dressed, her vocabulary, language, and accent when she speaks, her posture of confidence or submission, her friendship with someone in the clinic—all of these become part of the environment conditioning the relationship between service provider and client. These indicators of the client's identity are then interpreted through the lens of the service providers' official training. The population imperatives are intertwined with others on age, femininity, class, and others to shape the kinds of choices that service providers believe that women should make about methods and fertility control. For example, a service provider in a regional hospital, Mama Tanga explained that women are taught that four is the number of pregnancies that they can have safely [*kwa usalama*] but that any pregnancy above four is risky.[14]

Speizer et al. (2000) argue from survey data that Tanzanian service providers unnecessarily restrict access to contraceptive methods because their training and supervision is inadequate, but they also mention that providers' own norms and attitudes may be important. Even feminist health providers may "overlook subtle coercive or eugenicist public policies advanced by people with a political agenda of control of the reproduction of certain groups: low-income women, women of colour, and young women of all colours and classes" (Begus 1998, 221). While technologies are preconfigured for the generic, Western body, in the context of implementation, identity matters.

Women's Responses as Both Complying with and Countering Scattered Hegemonies

Planning one's family, through whatever means, has been a sign of disciplined bodies, upholding the social order and perpetuating values of self-control, restraint, and prudence.[15] Tanzanian women interviewed in clinics described both traditional and modern means for planning one's family. In most cases, women described the *njia za hospitali* [hospital based methods] first, and I had to follow up with a specific question about the existence of traditional methods. Almost a third of all respondents described a traditional method to me when I asked about ways that women could plan their families. These included calendar, mucus, withdrawal, external traditional methods like the *pigi*, internal traditional methods such as ingestible herbs, and abstinence. In ways similar to the discourses of international donors and of national level implementers, traditional family planning was talked about by women in two very different ways: as either a lost knowledge or as the indigenous equivalent to modern contraceptives. The language used and the needs articulated around all methods were the same. Women questioned the effectiveness and the side effects of all types of contraception. The identity issues for women appeared to be different than those for service providers: women saw modern identity as arising from the outcome, not the method choice itself.

Informants described how traditional practices emphasized this issue of discipline. Miriam, a 36-year-old mother of three living children answered my question of whether it was an embarrassment for a woman to have her children close together explaining, "Yes. It is a big shame to have your children one right after the other. You can't be respected in your community if this happens."[16] Miriam had the modern outcome of a well-spaced, well-planned family, yet she did not use the modern route for achieving it. The incompatibility between traditional methods and modern bodies was not described as a question of anachronism and loss of power, but one of ineffective service provision and poor quality of care on the part of the traditional healers. For example, one woman from a village in Morogoro Region explained:

> There are traditional methods of family planning, like roots to wear. However, they aren't very reliable. You can use them and not know if they are genuine. Some are just lies and are able to kill children. The traditional healers are just looking to make some money. They are all from Tanga [a different region]; none are from here.[17]

The issues of reliability and side effects, and even the idea of an imported, and therefore suspect, knowledge, come through in this sort of discussion of traditional methods.

The idea that a gap exists between the lost knowledge of traditional practices and the adoption of the new modern regimen as discussed by Tumbo-Masabo (1994) was also articulated by women whom I interviewed. For example, one respondent from a village where traditional methods of birthspacing based on postpartum abstinence were encouraged explained, "Nowadays, women have many children—more than in the past. Every year they have another child." She went on to describe how her own mother had waited until after three years before having another child, planning to space her births. In the opinion of some, usually older women, modern women are not as effective as the previous generations in spacing their children. So, like the government officials, these women are interested in this lost knowledge and in better disciplining of the younger generations. There is a sense of anachronism that while the traditional methods no longer work for modern bodies, the modern methods are not making the grade either.

Women's room for maneuver within the formal health care system was limited. From my observations, it seemed that women who came to clinics were aware of the correct stance on contraception, and if they deviated, it was by quietly not complying or by staying away from the clinic. Some women continued to use traditional methods, others used modern methods sporadically and for short periods of time, and still others used no family planning at all, a point to which chapter seven will return. Each instance of use or non-use of a method may provide women with a way of countering the expected dichotomy that traditional methods are for traditional bodies and modern ones for modern bodies. Yet the women who used them did not privilege one type of method over the other. One example comes from Asha, a 28-year-old woman who had used *dawa* [medicine] she received from an old woman who enclosed it in a cloth and tied it around her waist. She used this method in spacing the births of her first three children. After a miscarriage four years later, Asha decided to use pills. She said that she wanted to use them instead of the traditional methods because, as she explained:

> If you get bad traditional medicine, you can lose your ability to give birth completely. If you use the hospital methods and then something goes wrong, you can come back, and they can treat you. Therefore, it is better to use the hospital methods.[18]

Asha's description of how it is better to use modern methods in case there is any problem of side effects runs counter to the voices of other women who fear these methods specifically because of their side effects (Johnson-Hanks 2002; Russell, Sobo, and Thompson 2000, Rutenberg and Watkins 1997). It also calls into questions assumptions about the relationship between traditional healer and client. It shows that both types of methods are being considered in the same way, as strong technologies for intervening in one's reproductive process.

Some other women were using modern methods to circumvent, while appearing to uphold, traditional expectations of body discipline (see Bledsoe 2002). For example, a number of young women in Kanga, a village where modern family planning was not widely used, told me that they had used condoms. When I questioned the circumstances surrounding this choice, I found out that modern family planning was a literal replacement for a traditional method. In this community, women were expected to abstain for sexual relations during the postpartum period until the child was weaned. A young woman elaborated, "Condoms are good when nursing a child because the semen will spoil the breast milk." By using condoms, women were able to have the effect of having met the traditional expectations of their community while actually returning to sexual activity with their partners, and thus preventing a loss of power in this realm. Interestingly, it was the traditional expectation and belief that women described as driving their choices toward modern contraception.

The understanding of modern family planning for modern women with modern bodies and traditional methods as part of a traditional mindset as an obstacle to this identity did not make sense in the body practices of Tanzanian women. The outcome of planning one's family, usually articulated as not having births too close together, but also in some cases, as not having more children than you could care for, was more significant in women's self-described understanding of who was modern and who was not. However, the narrow focus of the family planning apparatus on limiting population growth made it more difficult, but not impossible, for women to make their own reproductive choices.

Conclusions

International politics, national policies, and local prejudices all interact in structuring relationships at local clinics. Sometimes countering and other times complying with the scattered hegemonies of the global population discourse, Tanzanian women as both service providers and clients must negotiate family planning. While Tanzanian women are pragmatic (see Lock and Kaufert 1998) in their reproductive strategies, their choices are also prearranged by nearby and distant discourses. A development apparatus creates problems, like overpopulation in a way that structures the kinds of interventions that are possible for their solution (see Ferguson 1994), yet these do not determine outcomes (see Cruikshank 1999).

New technologies have been interpreted through existing lenses of traditional family planning strategies. However, tradition itself is being brokered through the needs of legitimacy and modernity, as described earlier in the chapter as lost knowledge. This intellectual brokerage has proved particularly useful for both policymakers and service providers in attempts to translate the need for family planning interventions.

Notions of tradition and modernity are ubiquitous in such settings. We cannot understand contraceptive choice as taking place in isolation from the differing and contested notions of development. Women mixed methods and mixed messages in their practices of family planning, engaging in multiple forms of improvisation (see Tilly 1999). The entire dichotomy of traditional and modern constructed at other levels of the Tanzanian discourse on family planning did not make sense in the lives of women themselves. Material conditions in local clinics and in the lives of those who staff them intertwine with markers of identity; thus, family planning provides opportunities for enhancing material and symbolic capital at many levels. Service providers are caught between the prerequisites of modernity including higher contraceptive rates and the realities of dilapidated local clinics and uncooperative local bodies. This chapter has focused on the foot-soldiers of the family planning infantry and on the negotiation of technologies. The following chapter will examine how the recipients of the population discourse, Tanzanian women, and to some extent their partners, respond to the messages that they are receiving.

Intermezzo 3

Cost-Sharing and Bargaining in the Tanzanian Health Sector

One afternoon when we were driving out of the farm where we stay, we gave a ride to a woman and her child from the house. Along the roadside, we saw one of the young men who works in the yard of the landlord's house with a child on his back. The woman riding with us said that the child was sick. We stopped and asked them to get in the car. It seems that the child had started with a high fever, trembling and vomiting in the morning, and the mother had told her brother to carry the child to the main road to wait for transport. The mother was to meet him there and they were to go together to the regional government hospital in town known by the pseudonym Miti. We took them into the car and left a message that the mother should meet us at the hospital. I tried to think of a better hospital to take the obviously very sick child. I had worked in Miti in 1996 and knew that it is, like other Tanzanian government hospitals, very poorly equipped and staffed. Having made the mistake during a previous field stay of driving a woman to the local public regional hospital, attempting to ensure that she actually received care, and later hearing news that she had died quickly of meningitis after having been treated with only aspirin, I feared repeating the same scenario. Still, I did not know of any better option close by, and the mother was already planning to meet us at the Miti hospital. I decided to try to help the young child by taking him in and negotiating the procedures to get him basic care.

In policy, treatment of illness should be free for young children, but I know from experience that this is not the case in practice. Together with the young gardener, we took the child into the Miti reception. The first step was to understand where to start, even though I had spent months in the hospital before. The hospital is Byzantine, and without knowing exactly who to see first, you can spend hours waiting unnecessarily in the wrong line before being sent somewhere else. I introduced myself to the first uniformed nurse I saw, remembering to include the details that would help us to get proper service—that I was "Dr. Lisa Richey" and that I had worked at Miti Hospital in 1996. She kindly escorted us to the reception area where we began the process.

The two nurses at the reception were reluctant to admit the child because he had no notebook. At first, I thought that they meant that he was lacking the immunization record that is given during the monthly vaccinations and weighing. I found out after some discussion that it was not a *particular* notebook, but that he needed any notebook. Without one, the doctors could become *wakali sana* [very cross], they told me. I was able to pay the nurse who had brought us around to go just outside the entrance to a small stand to buy a basic school notebook for 200 Tsh. This provided the child's ticket to see the doctor. Again, at this point, I introduced myself extensively, even giving the doctor my business card to try to ensure that the child would be taken seriously and given the proper lab tests, particularly a malaria blood slide. The doctor agreed and sent the child to the lab. When I asked him if there were any fees to be paid, he was rather hesitant, perhaps because we both knew that official policy is that services for these children are free. He told me that he did not think that there were charges for young children, but that it was best that I go with them and ask at the lab. We all went to the lab, and indeed, there were no formal charges, but we had to pay 100 Tsh for a sterile lancet to prick his finger. I hesitate to think what they use for people who do not pay the fee. The lab technician gave us back the notebook with the child's results written inside. His parasite count was 200 out of 200 according to the handwritten note. I tried to understand if this was a mistake, as my own count with malaria two weeks before had been 2 out of 200, causing a lot of concern to my own doctor.

We returned, notebook in hand to Dr. Mapunda who said that indeed the child was very sick with malaria and his count was 200 parasites. He said that they would admit the child and start him on quinine. I asked if they ever used the Chinese artemisial derivative drugs here, since these are extremely effective and have far fewer side effects (having recently finished a course of them myself). Dr. Mapunda did not seem to know of them at all. Probably because at a cost of 6,000 Tsh per course, they would not have much opportunity to prescribe them to the strata of patients who come to Miti Hospital. I had gotten mine from a well-to-do pharmacist in the nearest major city who claimed that they were so expensive because they had to be imported from Belgium, and that he was the only one who had these connections. We had to call him out from a huge wedding celebration to retrieve the pills for me from his store on a Saturday, which might have incurred an additional processing fee. It was worth it to avoid another hospitalization with a quinine drip. From my own experience and many friends with malaria in Tanzania, I knew that quinine together with an antibiotic would cure the child, even as it was debilitating in the process, so I felt relieved that at least the doctor seemed to diagnose and prescribe an effective treatment from a layperson's perspective. I asked if the prescribed medicines were available in the hospital and the doctor laughed and said, "I don't know. Sometimes some are available and others are not. You will have to ask at the pharmacy." I also asked about payment for admission into the ward and was told predictably that I would have to ask at the ward itself. By this point, the child's mother had come with another female relative.

We all went to the ward to ask about admitting the child. The ward for children 4B consisted of one rectangular, cement room with dim electric lights, no window screens, and small dirty mosquito nets tied over single beds with sheet-less mattresses. On each bed were a minimum of two children and two female caregivers. Most children were hooked up to IV's and were lying motionless on the beds. One child was being held by his mother on the cement steps of the block, while the nurse used the natural light to help in inserting the IV needle into his tiny veins. He whimpered a bit, and his mother swatted at him, telling him to stop crying. It takes a lot of social conditioning in these children to build up the stoicism you see in adults here. We managed to talk with the nurse after she finished the insertion. She was visibly irritable and probably exhausted from having to deal with a ward that was obviously at least double the capacity of seriously ill children than it was supposed to be. When I showed her the list of drugs and supplies, she told the mother of the child that she could get them "perhaps tomorrow" [*labda kesho*]. I understood that this could mean that they would come the next day, some other day, or not at all. With a malaria count so high, the child would perhaps be dead by the next morning with no treatment. I asked if we could buy the supplies. The pharmacy was just outside the gate.

Mama Yusef, her month-old baby on her back, and I walked to the pharmacy. I gave them the list and they started to gather the supplies we needed. We had a problem with the glucose IV solution, as they seemed to be out of stock. The pharmacist directed Mama Yusef to another pharmacy down the street while I waited for the rest of the medicine. When Mama Yusef returned, she said that because it was nearly 6:00 pm on Sunday evening, the other pharmacy had closed. The retailer began to look a little harder to see if she had a bottle in one of the new stock boxes, yet to be shelved. Finally she told us that she had no half liter bottles but she had a full liter bottle. "Fine," I said, "We'll take it." The final count consisted of one vial of quinine (300 Tsh), one giving set for the IV (300 Tsh), one scalp vein needle (150 Tsh), one 2cc syringe (100 Tsh), one bottle of septrine (600 Tsh), and one bottle of dextrose glucose solution for IVs (1200 Tsh). They threw in two band-aids for free on account of our expensive order. We took the bag full of supplies back to the ward to discuss them with the nurse. She had ordered a half liter bottle and had to be seriously convinced that she could just throw out half of the contents of our bottle and have the same thing, thus starting the IV immediately. I tried to talk to Mama Yusef about bringing him food and boiled water, as they have nothing at the hospital. She could not stay with him, since she was caring for her one-month old baby, so the other relative would stay. When things seemed to be in order, I left.

On my way back from town at around 7:00 pm, I wanted to check to see if the IV had actually been inserted. From my experience, I know that the possibility was great that when I left, nothing had moved. Fortunately, when I checked in, Yusef was lying at the foot of a bed with his aunt and had been given the IV. He had a small bottle of solution, suggesting to me that the larger, and doubly expensive one had been pocketed for someone else's use, and that out of nowhere another half-liter bottle had materialized. None of the nets were over the beds, and with the small size beds full of four to six people, they could not have been much help anyway. The doors and windows were open, suggesting to me that anyone who did not already have malaria would be quite likely to get it while in the hospital. I went home. Later in the week, I asked for news of Yusef and heard only that his mother had gone down to the hospital to see him. Another week later, a man who appeared to be a farm worker knocked on my door in the evening. He was Yusef's father and had come to thank me for "saving the life of his son." Embarrassed and frustrated that it may indeed have taken a pushy white woman politely begging for assistance in Kiswahili to have gotten Yusef minimal care for a very common disease, I gave the standard reply, "your welcome—it was nothing."

6

Contraceptive Technologies for Planning Local Families

Introduction: The "Family" in Family Planning

The idea that contraception is for married women has long since fallen out of vogue in most of the Western discourse on reproductive health; in fact, the importance of access for adolescents to birth control has been a significant and highly contested component of implementing the post-Cairo reproductive health agenda. However, in many Third World countries contraceptives are still most often condoned only when they are used within the familial context. Even in a family planning program like India's, known for its rigor and outspoken criticism of high fertility, women are expected to be both modern and wifely. In describing how the national family planning program in India defines the modern Indian woman, Chatterjee and Riley explain "though they are represented as social agents capable of rational action and of improving their lives, contraception is never linked to unrestrained sexuality and seldom to nonfamilial roles" (2001, 832). An article by Cohen (2000) on the relationship between family planning service provision and contraceptive use by women in Malawi suggests that the family emphasis also shapes Malawian decision making. It concludes that the "most immediate need" is for reversible methods of modern contraception that can be used for child spacing, as most women report a desire to space births but not the stop childbearing completely (Ibid.). Thus, while the terms of the global discourse on reproductive health call for broadening the scope of family planning programs, in practice, these are still largely the domain of married couples planning for parenthood.

In response to the international paradigm shift from fertility control to promoting women's reproductive health, the National Family Planning Programme in Tanzania was renamed the National Reproductive and Child Health Programme. For some time, the significance in this seemed to be located in the relationship between the Tanzanian Ministry of Health and its international donors and lenders, and the questions that arose centered around the meaning and depth of such a paradigm shift for the way that family planning services, or reproductive health services, were promoted and provided at the local level. However, as I continued analyzing data from interviews with women and men around issues of family planning, a new question emerged. Why did they rename it the program on reproductive and *child* health?[1] Choosing to accentuate the continuity between interventions previously termed Maternal and Child Health/Family Planning (MCH/FP) in Tanzania may reflect the desire to maintain support and momentum built over years of overcoming resistance to population control measures, and it may also be a means of picking and choosing amongst the items promoted as the Cairo agenda.[2]

In this chapter, I argue that it also reflects what may be the most generalizable "local lens" for understanding family planning: in Tanzania, "family planning" focuses on having children, not on avoiding them. In cultures of childbearing, like those found in Tanzania, where deciding to opt out of having children is not really an option for women, the most important thing a contraceptive can do is to enable you to have healthy, well-provided for children. The conditions under which a pregnancy becomes auspicious are conditioned by discourses on gender, health, and modernity. The ubiquity of childbearing for adult women, the centrality of maintaining the health of the mother and her children, and the imperative to care for your children properly all shape the context of fertility decision making. These lenses also have implications for how various fertility technologies are perceived and used.

In describing the local lens through which the global population discourse and all of its constituent narratives are filtered, I shift my level of analysis to individual families. In doing so, I consider the local lenses of contraception that were related to me by Tanzanian women and men who live in a society were norms about fertility are changing, and contraceptives are used in ways that reflect diversity in reproductive desires, but emphasize the desire to reproduce. My ongoing research in Tanzania suggests that some women and their husbands may be using contraception to have fewer children while others use it to have more. However, the dynamics involved in planning one's family and choosing to use contraception look similar.

Contingency in Tanzania

As described earlier in the book, Tanzania was one of the first sub-Saharan African countries to offer family planning services in 1959, yet it was one of the last to declare an official national population policy in 1992. However, as argued in chapter three, its family planning program has been regarded as a success: contraceptive rates have increased and total fertility rates are declining. Yet, Tanzania still has lower levels of contraceptive use than expected when compared to other African countries with a similarly educated population (Lloyd, Kaufman, and Hewett 1999) and three-quarters of all married women are not using any form of family planning (Tanzania Bureau of Statistics, Planning Commission 2000). My interview data suggests that Tanzanians do not use contraception in the ways anticipated by the National Family Planning Programme, that is, contracepting for long periods of time to limit fertility. The discord between what Tanzanian women say about planning one's pregnancies, using contraception, and caring for one's children and the policy recommendations on fertility levels, birth intervals, and child health comes from the fact that a woman's self-defined "need" for family planning, and her ability to meet that need rarely converge.

It is not the case in Tanzania that women know about family planning, but are unwilling to use it, nor is it usually the case that they want to use contraception but lack access to modern methods. My data suggest that many women use modern family planning, but they do so for short periods of time and with limited success in meeting the ideal patterns of fertility promoted by national programs and their international funders (i.e., four children or less, born to mothers between the ages of 21 and 34, and spaced more than two years apart). Two recent works address such a possibility of a "regime of more sporadic birth control use" (Fisher and Szreter 2003) in the case of early-twentieth-century Britain, and (Johnson-Hanks 2002) in contemporary Cameroon. This chapter illustrates such a sporadic regime in the case of Tanzania, where reproductive decision making does not fit with notions of the fertility transition model—a calculus of conscious choice and parity-specific planning using biomedically efficient contraception (Johnson-Hanks, 2002)—however, in a case where fertility transition seems to be occurring nonetheless.

Tanzanian women do not seem to be for or against family planning—everyone knows about it, and while most know some side effects, they are still interested in using it when they perceive that the costs of getting pregnant are higher than those of using family planning. Tanzanian women do plan their families, but not often in the way that population control enthusiasts would like. Sometimes what women want is sex, but what they get is children. Other times, the desired goal is children, even to the point of planning a pregnancy alone and not telling the father. Children are not always desired in the sense of the traditional value of children, and some women faced with an unwanted pregnancy try to abort. Not surprisingly, no single theory of reproductive intentions seems to fit with the realities of women's lives. Sometimes some factors take precedence, while other times the parameters of decision making are different. Still other times, women plan one thing, but actually get a different outcome. Context is critical in understanding reproductive decision making and thus, this chapter attempts to shed light on some of the contextual factors that constitute the most relevant lenses for contraceptive technologies.

My reading of local Tanzanian women's responses to population policy through family planning interventions draws insight from Bledsoe's (2002) work in The Gambia. Bledsoe assembles and elaborates on the many challenges presented by women in The Gambia to standard notions of fertility and contraception. Gambian reproduction is linked not to a time-based notion of senescence where the body is given a certain number of years between menarche and menopause to reproduce, but to "a God-given endowment that must be realized within a life course of contingent physical tolls" (Ibid., 212). The entire discourse of childbearing in The Gambia differs greatly from that of Western-based fertility studies, but perhaps less from the actual reproductive experiences of Western women. Still, Bledsoe notes:

> The fact that an entire segment of what rural West Africans see as the "normal" female physical life course simply does not exist in the United States is a remarkable commentary on the role of social life in shaping cultural perceptions of the body's "natural" temporalities (Ibid.).

The social contingency of bodies is an important part of understanding the impasse between global discourse and local realities. Bledsoe finds that Gambian women are using highly effective modern contraceptives to rest and regain capacity, often after experiencing a reproductive mishap (miscarriage, stillbirth, or death of an infant): contraceptives are used to enable Gambian women to have more children, not fewer.

Local discourses always linked to other discourses, including the international discourse on reproductive health that promotes family planning as a means of realizing women's reproductive rights. Also, a focus on the family in family planning can be found at all levels of implementation of population policy in Tanzania, and has shaped the national level interpretation of the population problem as one of quality, not quantity as I describe in chapter two. It has also provided legitimacy under which the UMATI [*Uzazi na Malezi Bora*] has supplied the country with contraception since 1959 as outlined in chapter four. For example, an UMATI report explicitly uses such justification: "UMATI has repeatedly emphasized the fact that its goal is not to spread family planning for the purpose of population control but rather to enable families to have healthier children and to protect the health of the mother and ultimately the whole family will be healthy and lead a happy life" (Kihamia and Maro 1984, I).

While this chapter examines what I understand as a local lens, it is worth remembering that discourses are always read in relation to other discourses such as the global and national ones described in the first section of the book. Simply identifying and deconstructing a development discourse does not destroy its legitimacy (Cooper and Packard 1997) and conversely, describing a local discourse as such does not legitimate it over other discourses. Following on from chapters five and six, this chapter continues exploring the intersections between abstract, generic plans of the global population discourse and small-scale social life.

My discussion draws on Bledsoe's use of contingency, which together with the concept of cumulativity, is central to understanding reproduction within a woman's life course. Contingency is particularly relevant for understanding fertility control in Tanzania because it emphasizes the fact that circumstances, not time or some target number of children, pose the limits on wanting more pregnancies or children (Ibid., 212). Thus, in societies where high fertility is the goal, women's fertility decision making is based on the circumstances surrounding the potential that a pregnancy will result in a healthy birth; thus, women try to maximize the utilization of their reproductive potential to deliver as many healthy babies, born in auspicious social settings, as possible.

This lens for viewing the contextuality of fertility in light of the contingency of the life course is compelling, and may be useful even in understanding societies like Tanzania where high fertility is no longer always the goal, although for some women it still is. Here I would argue that the circumstances likely to lead to the desire for a pregnancy are likely to conform to a slightly expanded, yet somewhat more rigid criteria, before a pregnancy becomes truly "planned." Higher aspirations for one's offspring, shaped by spiraling "expectations of modernity" to borrow Ferguson's term (1999), contribute an additional layer of conditionality that must be met before childbearing is deemed auspicious. Thus, it may be that the processes are the same for thinking about fertility decision making between Gambian women and Tanzanian women; however, the assessment of when the context may be ripe for another child varies around contingencies of bodily depletion as described by Bledsoe, and also social and economic viability of taking care of a new child together with one's existing children.

The following section discusses the relationship between notions of planning, implementation of plans, pregnancy, and children. The next sections analyze specifically cases of unwanted pregnancy, and planning for after one has begun childbearing. Then the penultimate section considers the special case of Kilimanjaro Region, a community experiencing fertility transition. The last section draws some conclusions on the context of planning, pregnancy, and contraceptives. In spite of the fact that this chapter focuses on when women have used contraception, it is important to remember that at the time of any given survey so far, most Tanzanian women are *not* using contraception.[3] As Warwick reminds us, " the fact that some women go to heroic lengths to limit their fertility does not negate the fact that many do not" (Warwick 1982, 36). Drawing on the existing family planning literature, we would expect to be able to broadly characterize Tanzanian women of reproductive age as: 1) not willing to use modern family planning because of attitudinal reasons such as fear of side effects, or traditional mindsets toward having many children and not controlling fertility or 2) as a vast pool of women with unmet need, desperately seeking to limit their fertility and/or space their pregnancies, but without a means to do so. However, my research has found that Tanzanian women who attend MCH/FP clinics were relatively well-informed about modern family planning, and often used it to meet their contextually defined needs of fertility regulation. Therefore, women who were not currently using contraception were not likely to oppose its usage either—as one woman from a remote village told me when I asked if people approved of family planning:

> People agree! They have so many children—one here, one there—they can't even go to the fields. They agree with family planning now. Services are available. There is no problem to get it (Interview 10716).

However, as many studies have confirmed, knowledge and approval[4] do not necessarily translate into using family planning in the ways promoted by the population discourse—contracepting for long periods of time to limit fertility.

Planning, Pregnancy, and Children

Mtoto umleavyo ndivyo akuavyo *[As you bring up a child, so does he grow up]*

—a well-known Kiswahili proverb

I expected that drawing a sample of non-users would produce respondents who fit broadly into three categories: 1) women who had never used contraception because they disagreed with it either categorically or specifically, that is, regarding side effects; 2) women who had used contraception in the past, but had experienced problems with it, and thus were unwilling to continue; and 3) women who were not using contraception because they wanted to conceive.[5] However, one of the most surprising results of this work was that most women (76 percent) in the entire sample had indeed used contraception.[6] Of my sample of current non-users of family planning, half (n=51) had been users in the past. Table 6.1 shows the methods chosen by these women during their reproductive history of contraceptive use. Note that the total sample is more than the total number of women interviewed as each use of a different method is counted, so a single woman may have used three methods at different points in her reproductive history. As always, there may be problems of recall, especially for older women who may have used numerous methods during their reproductive histories. However, there are not problems of multiple method use where women used more than one method simultaneously, because the interview narratives were sensitive to this possibility, but it was not actually discussed. In the following discussion, the percentages shown are to compare the popularity of the methods used by women.[7]

Table 6.1 Methods Ever Used by Sampled Tanzanian Women

Methods Ever Used	*Percentage of All Methods Used by Women*			
	Total Sample n=200	*Morogoro Region n=120*	*Ruvuma Region n=40*	*Kilimanjaro Region n=40*
Pill	37.9	38.4	42.2	32.7
Depo-Provera	22.9	20.5	17.8	34.7
Condom	22.9	28.8	20.0	8.2
Calendar/Rhythm	3.8	0.7	4.4	12.2
Norplant	3.8	6.2	0.0	0.0
IUD	2.9	1.4	2.2	8.2
Sticks/String/*Pigi*	2.1	1.4	6.7	0.0
Female Sterilization	1.7	0.7	4.4	2.0
Abstinence	1.3	0.7	2.2	2.0
Foam/Tablets	0.8	1.4	0.0	0.0
Mucus	0.0	0.0	0.0	0.0
Withdrawal	0.0	0.0	0.0	0.0
Male Sterilization	0.0	0.0	0.0	0.0
Herbs/Ingested	0.0	0.0	0.0	0.0
Diaphragm	0.0	0.0	0.0	0.0
Other	0.0	0.0	0.0	0.0
Total	100.0	100.0	100.0	100.0

Source: Interviews with the Author.

Of women who had ever used family planning (n=150), most began using the pill (45 percent) as their first method. As the most consistently available modern method in Tanzania, and one that is promoted in clinics, this would be expected. Interestingly, the second most popular method for first-time family planning was condoms (27 percent).[8] The popularity of condoms as the first family planning method used speaks to the importance of male involvement in contraception, and to the willingness of African couples to tolerate the inconveniences of "short-term" contraception—something we would not expect from the portrayal of condoms in the clinic setting or from the global population discourse. It may also reflect awareness and practice of HIV/AIDS and sexually transmitted disease prevention. Some women said that the reason they had chosen to use condoms was to prevent sexually transmitted diseases; these were also women who described using condoms with a man who was not their partner.[9] For example:

> Amina, 22 years old, described how she had used condoms as her first method of family planning for 9 months before she was "together" with her husband. She said that she used them to protect herself from both

> STDs and pregnancy. She was the one who decided to use the condoms, but her partner agreed and he liked them. She stopped using them after moving in with her husband because they wanted her to get pregnant.[10]

While condoms were popular as the first methods of family planning used, the link between condoms and prevention of STDs made the use of condoms after developing a relationship or marriage a much more difficult issue. In Kilimanjaro Region, where AIDS awareness was already high and its impact was talked about in local communities,[11] two women brought up the constraints they faced regarding the use of condoms within their marriages. The following passage is from my reflections after having interviewed these two women:

> Two women were forthcoming in talking about their fears of contacting AIDS from their husbands. One woman, a 38-year-old farmer, told me that she is careful for herself, and does not have any extramarital sexual partners, but she doesn't know what her husband does. She said that she asked him to use a condom if he goes with other women, but he refuses. She asked me about ways to protect herself, and I told her that if she is unable to be sure of her husband, then she needs to use a condom with him. She agreed, but said that he would refuse because it would incriminate him as someone who is sleeping around. She said that he knows that she is using Depo-Provera, so he won't believe that condoms are for birth control. I suggested that she tell him that the Depo is giving her problems, so she has stopped taking it, while continuing to use it in secret. Then, perhaps she can convince him to use condoms, as he doesn't want any more children. Another woman, 50 years old and still subject to pregnancy, which she would not want at this point, expressed many of the same sentiments. She said that she knew many people who have died of AIDS, and she thinks there is no other illness like it. She said, "I don't know what my husband does—if he is sleeping around, there is no way for me to know." She told me that she is just leaving things up to God, as she feels helpless to do anything about it.[12]

The fears expressed by these two women, both of whom were empowered enough to use family planning, but not able to protect themselves from HIV/AIDS, illustrate some of the critical areas of women's reproductive health that lie fully outside of a narrow concentration on contraceptive use. On a different level, these also suggest that men may be willing to use condoms for pregnancy prevention within marriage, but not to prevent sexually transmitted diseases, which would label them as promiscuous.

My erroneous view, drawn from the literature at the time, was that Tanzanian women who used contraception would be somehow "different" from those who did not. However, Bledsoe (1994, 2002) describes how rural users are not a discrete group with characteristics that set them apart from non-users, but are instead "the crest of a moving wave of numerous temporary users who are simply using contraceptives for small slices of time during the birth interval if they find that their fecundity resumes too soon" (2002, 97). These are women who are trying to postpone the next pregnancy "as they juggle the conflicting demands of husbands and mothers-in-law and the health of their children" (Ibid.).

Similarly, in Tanzania, family planners of traditional and modern methods, and those we would label as "diligent" versus "noncompliant" users, all were using methods for analogous reasons: to take care of their health and the children they had already borne. In my interviews with women, I asked those who said that they had ever used family planning, why they decided to use it at that time. Exactly half of the women (67 out of 135 contraceptive users) responded that they chose to use contraception because of their existing child or children. Sara[13] from a village in Ruvuma had a baby boy a little over a year old when I interviewed her. She had given birth to a daughter three years earlier, but the baby died at around six months from "too little blood," a condition that Sara attributed to malaria. She began using contraceptive pills when her son Salim began to walk. At this point she resumed sexual relations with her husband, and went to the local health center for pills because she had friends who used them without problems. She explained: "I wanted to bring up my child so he will grow up well. Before, I didn't think that I could get pregnant."

Most of the women interviewed explained their use of family planning as a response to motherhood articulating their own versions of the well-known Kiswahili proverb that introduced our discussion: "as you bring up a child, so does she grow up." Sara told me that she would indeed like to have another child, "when Salim is three years old or even later." Another example comes from Aikande who explained: "I wanted to space my children, to take care of them" [*Nilipenda kuza watoto kwa mpangalio, kuwahudumia*.] The difference between the forms of the verb *kupanga* seems interesting, as Aikande is not really saying what we would translate into "planning" but using a word, *pangalio*, that is used to indicate "interposition, succession, alternation, rotation."[14] *Kupanga* would imply arranging births in a linear order as most demographic models suggest, while *kupangalia* has a reference more toward interposing births. Whether this is a conscious linguistic choice to signify "planning for" as opposed to simply "planning" in the abstract, I have no way to know; however, it may be pointing to a local lens of family planning that is highly contextualized in relation to Aikande's own assessment of the best way to care for her children. Family planning is not ordering one's fertility in accordance with a Platonic abstract of the "ideal number of children" but a process of ongoing decision making, based on life's contingencies.

The second part of Aikande's explanation may also shed some meaning on her decision-making process, when she says that she wants to "take care of them" [*kuwahudumia*] the use of the word implies serving or waiting on someone. Thus, she may be suggesting a particular kind of parenting, one that is labor-intensive for the caregiver. This is different than the more commonly heard expression for taking care of children [*kuwatunza*]. Without overinterpreting the issue, Aikande may lend support to Caldwell's theories of fertility transition that come when the wealth flows shift away from children supporting parents, to parents serving their children. Thus, when parents are involved in waiting on their children, they may not want to have more than one resource-intensive child in the household at a time.[15]

Because the issues surrounding pregnancies are crucial for understanding women's ideas about their fertility choices, I talked with women about their first pregnancy and about the most recent pregnancy they had conceived by the time of our interview. I asked particularly about the first pregnancy, as it marked the onset of childbearing, and as such a significant change in one's lifecycle, may have entailed a different set of decision-making factors, and perhaps more or less planning than later pregnancies. I asked about the most recent pregnancy as a way of understanding the differences between this later pregnancy and the first one. My choice of first and most recent pregnancies was also based on the expectation that these conceptions may be more likely to have been unplanned and would bring up discussions of family planning and understanding more about unwanted pregnancies.[16] Because I had also taken an entire history of all conceptions that the women could recall, I was able to place these discussions in the larger context of the woman's pregnancy history.

The general tendencies from my sample show that first and most recent pregnancies were most often to women who married the fathers,[17] and who were not trying to get pregnant, but nonetheless, considered their first child to have been "wanted." Zainabu gave what represents a typical description:

> I felt glad. It just happened. I wasn't using anything to try not to get pregnant, but I wasn't upset that it happened. The father was happy. [They got married later in the same year when she was 18].

Zainabu links her pregnancy to her relationship with the child's father, and while she was not actively pursuing pregnancy, she was not preventing it either. Like most women in my sample, Zainabu began her childbearing in her late teenage years,[18] engaging in "high-risk" reproductive practices as defined by the global population discourse,[19] but in "normal" reproductive behavior according to Tanzanian norms.

Unlike the clear distinctions drawn by large-scale surveys where desire for children is measured as a dichotomous variable (i.e., the pregnancy was wanted or unwanted), my research shows that there is a very blurry line between when a pregnancy is actually wanted or not. Getting women to talk about their feelings, including desires, expectations or plans, at the time when they found out that they were pregnant was difficult. For example, some women, when I asked them about how they felt, told me that they had felt nauseous or dizzy. When I probed further about whether they had been glad about the pregnancy or whether they had planned, I received mixed responses. Respondents commonly told me that pregnancies were not planned, but that they were happy that they had gotten pregnant. When I asked women how they felt when they knew that they had become pregnant, some women said that they were simply "surprised." Many women told me that getting pregnant was just "typical" [*ya kawaida*]—something that just happens to women. When Maria first became pregnant, she said "it just happened" [*ilitokea tu*]. She said that she "had a few minor symptoms" but she was happy—"it was a typical thing." She told me that she did not plan it, "but once it had happened I was glad—what else?" The father was happy—"Perhaps he planned it" she mused. Pregnancy in this context is very much part of gendered identity of femaleness: it is an expected state as part of normal life.[20]

Most women (57 percent) said that they were happy with their first pregnancy, whether or not they were already married. For women and men who were married, the first pregnancy was universally welcomed. The notion of delaying the onset of childbearing for any reason, once a couple was married, did not make sense in the context

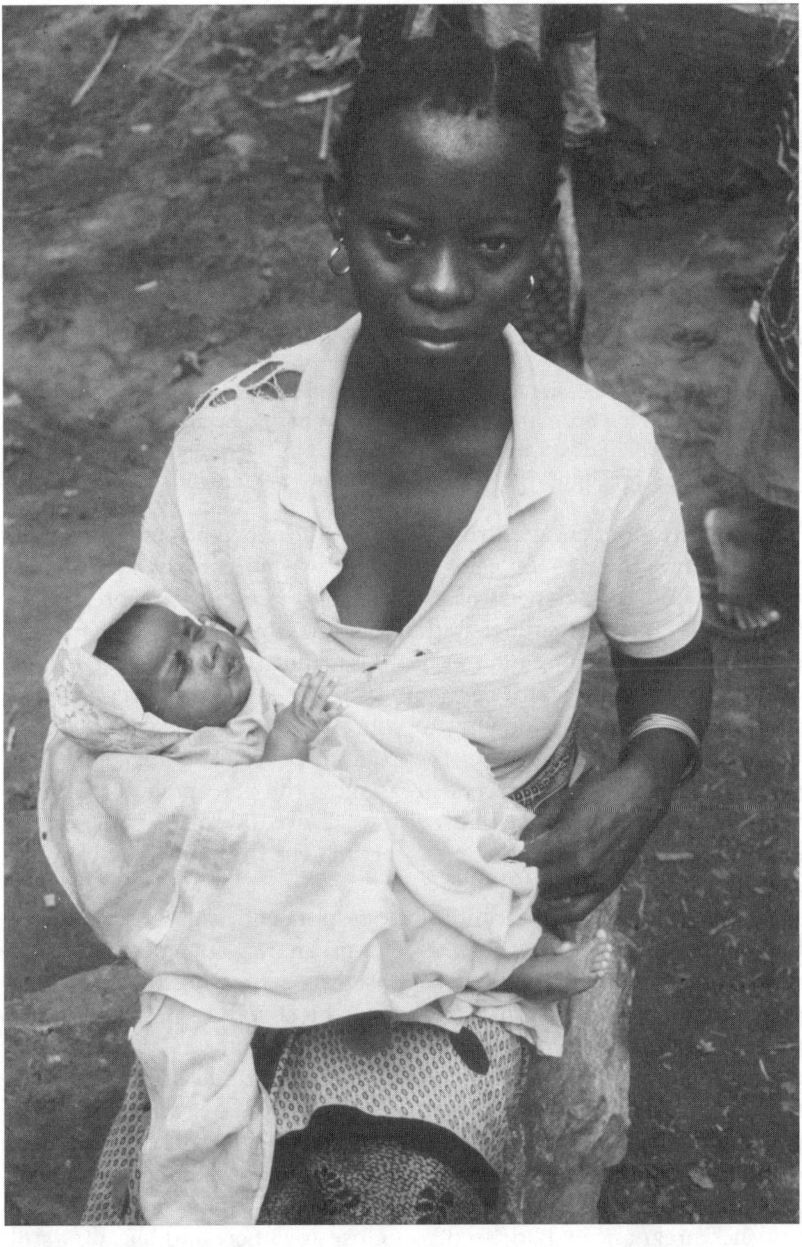

Photo 7 A Young Mother Poses with Her New Infant

Source: Photograph by Lisa Ann Richey.

described by women. For example, Rosina told me: "I had married a man so it was necessary that I have a pregnancy!" [*Nimeolewa na bwana, lazima mimba iwe*!].

Half of my respondents linked the reason that they were happy to be pregnant the first time with the fact itself that they were married. Some respondents who were married expressed relief at conceiving their first pregnancy because of the high expectations that married women be fertile. Marriage in Tanzania is nearly synonymous with childbearing, and a delay in conceiving the first child can raise fears of infertility and threaten the marriage. For example, when I asked how she felt about her first pregnancy, Gertruda said:

> I had been married already for two years so I was glad to get pregnant. My husband felt normal [*ya kawaida*]—but he had been worried when we had been married a year without a child. He was afraid that I couldn't get pregnant! [She was 18 at the first pregnancy].

While this respondent was from a village, the expectation that women would bear children soon after marriage was not simply a rural phenomenon. Of all women interviewed about their first pregnancy (n=194), 47 percent said that they were trying to get pregnant: 37 percent had been trying for a year or less, and 10 percent had tried for over a year. One indicator of the importance of the first pregnancy is that of those who were trying to conceive, 11 percent were using a form of traditional medicine to promote conception for their first pregnancy. By the most recent pregnancy, the percentage of women using traditional medicine in order to conceive dropped to only 6 percent, suggesting that proving one's fertility the first time may be more important than ongoing childbearing.

While over half (52 percent) of the respondents said that they were happy to conceive their most recent pregnancy, the percentage of women who were unhappy, as opposed to expressing feeling somewhere in between, was much higher for most recent pregnancies (32 percent as compared to 17 percent for first pregnancies). Similarly, as described by the women, the percentage of their husbands who were unhappy with the pregnancy rose from only 4 percent with first pregnancies to 22 percent with the most recent pregnancy. One respondent, Semeni, explained that she had not planned her most recent pregnancy. It just happened by "bad luck" [*bahati mbaya*]. She said her pregnancies had been too close together, and she was still nursing the previous child. But Semeni's husband consoled her saying "this is the work of God."

Unwanted Pregnancies, Wanted Children?

Respondents were surprisingly frank about discussing when a pregnancy was completely unwanted. Out of 340 pregnancies in 200 respondents, 10 instances were described as having been abortions, attempted abortions, or seriously considered abortions.[21] I suspect that this number is an underestimate as women may have felt uncomfortable talking about their experiences with abortion, which is illegal in Tanzania except to save the mother's life. Still, from informal conversations I learned that many women have some idea about where one would go to receive an abortion if they needed it, even if most of my informants expressed disapproval of such actions. However, the following examples shown in table 6.2 were brought up during my gathering of a reproductive health history[22] of each woman.

Table 6.2 Pregnancy Outcomes Desired

	First Pregnancy	*Most recent Pregnancy*[a]
Considered Abortion	1	2
Attempted Abortion	1	2
Aborted	2	2
Total	4	6

Source: Original Data.

Note: [a]In the case of only one pregnancy, it is considered as "first pregnancy" and not also as "most recent pregnancy" to avoid double counting.

While I believe these numbers are an underestimate, because women are reluctant to discuss the issue of abortion,[23] I do think that the increase in clearly unwanted pregnancies between the first and most recent pregnancy is important, and coincides with the previous data about women's and men's feelings about the pregnancies.

Some women were clear that they did not want another pregnancy at the time they conceived, but once they had the child, they were glad. Latifa, age 38, said of her most recent pregnancy, her sixth child: "I was happy because God had given me a baby, but what could I do? I hadn't planned it. I had tried to take pills but because of my stomach problems, I had to stop them." Here the distinction clarified by Bledsoe (2002) between wanting a pregnancy and wanting a living, healthy child may help to clarify situations like Latifa's. In this case, the mother had planned not to have a pregnancy, but in retrospect, when the pregnancy resulted in a healthy baby from God, being happy seemed the only reasonable response.

The increase in the number of pregnancies that were to some degree unwanted may reflect previous experiences in childbearing and childrearing. More unwanted pregnancies may relate to a change in the perception on the basis of experience—that is, before having the first child, parents may have imagined the benefits but not the costs of children. Thus, these parents would find later pregnancies unwanted as they come to perceive having children as more difficult. Alternatively, more unwanted births after the first may also reflect a worsening of circumstances of the woman or couple over time. It may be the case that later-born children, coming into a family where other children are already present, are seen as more of a burden than earlier ones.[24] It also seems to suggest, unsurprisingly, that unlike the depiction of the traditional mindset where every African child is wanted, Tanzanians' fertility preferences are nuanced and responsive to the particularities of their life contexts.

While 55 percent of the women said that they were not trying to conceive with the most recent pregnancy, and 53 percent were not trying to conceive with the first child, the number of women who were using any method of family planning in order to prevent pregnancy at the time of their most recent conception was 16 percent as compared to only 3 percent with the first pregnancy. These data suggest that while women who conceived at a time when they were not planning to do so was similar for both first and most recent pregnancies, more women were using family planning as a method to prevent this conception for the most recent birth.[25] This gap between women who used family planning when conceiving the first child and those who used it when conceiving the most recent one is not surprising if we read it through the perspective that family planning, is most often understood to mean planning rest *after* a pregnancy. Thus, it should not be surprising that most women would not have begun using any family planning before the birth of their first child.

Planning After You Have a Family

The local lens that family planning is for women who already have children also shapes service provision in the National Family Planning Programme, making it difficult for women who are young, unmarried, or childless to be considered legitimate clients. Speizer et al. (2000) point out that service providers in Tanzanian clinics regularly impose restrictions on family planning usage on the basis of age, marital status, and parity. According to their quantitative study, barriers imposed by individual service providers that are based neither on government policy nor on medical justifications are restricting access to contraceptives, particularly for the important target population of adolescent women (Ibid.). However, another interpretation of these barriers is that they represent family planning as viewed through a local lens in Tanzania, one that integrally links contraception with childbirth. While the government policy and national guidelines for service provision reflect the priorities of the global population discourse as described in chapter four, the actual distribution of contraceptives at the clinic level relies equally on local discourses. In the international and national context, any woman has the right to use contraceptives; however in most local discourses, family planning becomes a consideration only after you have already begun to have a family.

One example of the local lens of need comes from the story of Isha, a woman interviewed in an urban clinic: Isha got pregnant for the first time at age 16 when she was traveling with her sister. When I asked how she felt about it, she said "just fine" [*safi tu*], but that it was unplanned. She was not using any form of family planning at the time. The father said that it was not his child and claimed that he had not done anything. Isha got help from her older sister and now lives with her child in her parents' house. When I asked her what she thought about family planning, she responded quite positively that "anyone at all can use family planning" and she explained to me "they use it not to get pregnant too quickly [for spacing]." For herself, however, she said, "I have no need for it, but after my child is two and is no longer breastfeeding, I will come in for family planning so as not to get pregnant too soon." At the time of our interview, Isha was relying on a combination of what may have been postpartum amenorrhea and abstinence, or at least not taking on a steady relationship, while her child was still nursing.[26] When I asked her why she had never used contraception in the past, she responded: "Before, I had no children, so I had no need for family planning." When you have no children, you have no need for family planning, even if you are having sexual activity and do not want a pregnancy. Despite having no help from the father of her child, when she had given birth to a healthy child, Isha was glad to have gotten pregnant. She had the support of her female family members and did not suggest that male support was an important consideration for her family planning decision making.[27]

While husband's or partner's support is not necessary for women to use family planning,[28] women who used contraception tended to do so with the agreement and approval of the men in their lives. For women who had ever used family planning, 59 percent decided together with their partner to initiate contraception and 72 percent said that their partner approved of their contraceptive method.[29] There is a contrast between what women say they actually did, usually involving partner support, and general expressions of female ingenuity in the face of male disapproval of contraception. In-depth interviews with couples, which I will describe in detail later in this chapter, suggest that it often happens that wife and husband will agree that they should do something for family planning, but then the wife, together with the clinic service provider, will decide what kind of method to use. While women report that men usually approve of the method they use, individual interviews suggest that men are not always completely clear on the specifics of their wives' method choice. Also, this picture of male approval does not necessarily contradict the popular perception that men are against contraception. During my observations at a Kilimanjaro clinic in 2000, service provides attributed the consistently increasing popularity of Depo-Provera as a result of secret usage by women with disapproving [*wakali*] husbands. However, Bledsoe suggests, "a man may give a negative answer, vehemently expressed and intensely meant, to an abstract query about his objections to family planning" (2002, 205). Yet, if his wife is unwell, or in the Tanzanian case, if the household circumstances are not conducive to a pregnancy, a man will be likely to produce a different, more contextually specific response.

When family planning is used in the context of marriage for child-spacing, it seems that most often both husbands and wives are involved in decision making. One illustrative example comes from in-depth interviews conducted separately with Mr. and Mrs. Edward at their home in Machame, Kilimanjaro Region. Their responses provide some insight into the meaning of contingent decision making on fertility in a specific conjugal context.[30] The Edwards live in a small cement house on the potholed, dirt road that leads to the village government clinic. The family is relatively poor for this community, but they were very interested in discussing their aspirations for the family, and particularly emphasized that their hopes lie in education for their children. Mama Edward had three living children (aged ten, eight, and four), and had given birth to another child who died shortly after birth. After her first child reached six months, she went to the local government clinic for pills. After having problems with high blood pressure, the nurses advised her to switch so she used an IUD until her husband had problems with it, so she stopped and had her second child. After that, Mama Edward switched to the injection. She hoped to have five or six children, because she told me, "if you have only a few, three or four, some can die."

Baba Edward told me that he and Mama Edward were married in 1990, the only marriage for each of them, and they had their first child in the same year. After this child, Baba and Mama Edward decided together to use family planning, but then she went alone to the clinic for advice.[31] Baba said that she switched to injections as advised at the clinic and that he planned to continue using them until they want another child. He said that whether or not to have another one would depend on the conditions of their life [*hali ya maisha*]. If things got better, then he might like another one. Life had become more difficult for the Edward family because he had once been the driver for the head of the region, but he lost his job in cutbacks in 1995 and now must survive by farming and selling his labor on others' farms. He would like for his children to have a modern life, including education up to Form 6 [secondary school] in a good school and nice clothes and healthy food. He discussed with me that probably he would *not* want another child, but he would decide together with his wife as they decide for other decisions around the family.

In sum, we cannot really claim that Baba and Mama Edward are in agreement or disagreement about their preferred family size. Together they will weigh the benefits of having more children as an insurance against Providence versus the costs of children in an economically trying time. The National Family Planning Programme, geographically only a couple of hundred meters away in the local MCH clinic, enters the Edwards' calculus of decision making through the provision of method options for situations of male discomfort or female contraindication to a particular method. However, as described in the previous chapter, service providers also provide advice and example on how falling pregnant can affect the conditions of life, and what kinds of expectations are modern for one's children. The Edwards' descriptions of their experiences with family planning represent general trends throughout both phases of my research: family planning was something that became relevant after giving birth to a child; when problems were encountered with contraception, advice was sought and strategies were changed; husband and wife communicated about these decisions, although the extent of such communication varied and its scope was partial; and overall, decision making was circumstantial, not essential, and both, how to plan childbearing and the means used to do so were issues for discussion, not dictation or divination.

However, some women decided to use contraception secretly when they were unable to agree with their partners about the desire for a pregnancy or the pace of childbearing. In my interviews, 14 percent of women were using contraception secretly, and another 3 percent were using it even though their husband knew and disapproved. For example, Mwanahamisi who came from Kanga, a remote village where family planning use was low, but services were available, lowered her voice when her husband was out of earshot and explained her situation. She told me that when she conceived her eighth pregnancy, "We had just become tired of having children! [*tumeshachoka kuzaa*!] It just happened, but his father was happy." After the eighth child was born, she went to the village clinic for Depo-Provera. She was using it secretly because her husband would not allow it—she said "Men want more children—men don't get tired!" However, when I asked her about the future, if she would like to have more children, she said, "Maybe in the future, maybe I would have two more, even five!" but she continued in contrast saying "I have already tired out, and I have already become old" (she was 41).

Many women, like Mwanahamisi, emphasized that men are in favor of large families because they do not feel the responsibility of caring for these children.[32] One respondent summed up men's position on childbearing when I asked her if her husband was glad when she had conceived her first pregnancy. She told me that *of course* her husband was glad: "Where you have planted your seeds, you intend to reap the harvest!" [*unapopanga mbegu zako, utategemea kuvuna*!].

The provision of contraceptives through the National Family Planning Programme provided opportunities for some women to become "disorderly" in evading their husbands' control, yet whether women were actually able to exploit these opportunities to achieve their own goals was linked to a variety of processes at the technological and social levels. This complexity is shown by the following example from a woman interviewed in an urban Moshi clinic. Abibi described what happened when she found that she disagreed with her husband over the timing of births and the use of family planning:

> Abibi started using contraceptive pills after the birth of her second child. She told me that she hid them from her husband because he did

> not approve of her using them at that time. He wanted her to give birth to five children and then stop altogether. When she saw that her fertility returned quickly between her first and second child, she said, "I used my craftiness" to take the pills. However, she began having problems with continuous menstrual bleeding and she stopped the pills. She said that she knew that she would get pregnant again, but that it was better than the problems she got from the pills.[33]

Abibi's case illustrates how difficult it can be for women to decide to use contraceptives and then to actually succeed in doing so. As Watkins, Rutenberg, and Wilkinson show for the case of Kenya, "even if a woman feels she should space or stop childbearing, and her husband agrees, there is a subsequent hurdle . . . whether 'white man's medicine rhymes with black women's bodies'" (1997, 234).

Reproductive Decision-Making Perspectives from Kilimanjaro

The previous sections of the chapter have characterized the lenses of contraception as intimately linking family planning with families, that is, having already had one or more children who constitute a family. The negotiations between partners around fertility, the centrality of child and maternal health, and the ubiquity of childbearing all support Bledsoe's (2002) analysis of Gambian society where fertility is contingent. However, in her analysis, Gambian women are using contraceptives to have as many children as possible, and Tanzania has experienced an unprecedented drop in fertility levels over the past decade. What do these inconsistencies mean for a contingent reading of fertility decision making?

This section will look at how these issues are being interpreted by married couples in a Tanzanian community that is on the forefront of fertility transition. Not surprisingly, this community is relatively affluent with greater numbers of public and private health care facilities, but it is also highly stratified at the household level with vast socioeconomic inequality. Thus, the randomly selected survey respondents should reflect a diverse spectrum of household economic situations all of whom are responding to the same types of policy interventions in the forms of similar community-level access to family planning. The Chagga of Tanzania seem to be on the forefront of the country's demographic transition. Kilimanjaro Region in Tanzania, and the Machame area in particular, are known as affluent Chagga communities. Indeed, as elaborated by Setel (1995, 1999), the Chagga are known reputationally as "East Africa's 'moderns.'" Howard (1994) points out that Kilimanjaro has more health and educational facilities and other signs of development than any other region in Tanzania. Similarly, the Chagga are overrepresented in both secondary and tertiary educational institutions, senior business and management positions, and the civil service. However, in spite of the affluence of the Chagga, government medical statistics show that the Kilimanjaro region has significantly higher rates of child malnutrition than poorer regions of the country (Howard 1994, 239). Chagga society on the mountain has become highly stratified, with huge differences developing between rich and poor, and between and among men and women (Mercer 1999, 203).[34] Aspirations of education are also becoming increasingly difficult to attain (see Vavrus 2003).

As mentioned previously, I followed the earlier three-region study of women with a second study on fertility decision making between married couples in Kilimanjaro Region. While I had been initially reluctant as a Western woman to interview Tanzanian men about fertility issues,[35] my earlier study suggested that most family planning was still confined to marriage relationships and men were an important part of this decision making. In the Machame area of Kilimanjaro, male and female assistants and myself interviewed married husbands and wives in approximately 250 randomly selected households.[36] I conducted follow-up in-depth interviews with a purposive selection of 10 households. As described above, Machame as a community is not representative of rural Tanzania as a whole, but presents us with a best case scenario for examining Tanzanian attitudes where fertility is on the decline and where facilities are available, socioeconomic indicators are strong, but at the same time, the level of economic inequality between different households is high. Most of the respondents had completed primary school, and a significant percentage had secondary education or more (see fig. 6.1). Machame residents are much better educated than other Tanzanians (nearly 42 percent of whom have received no education at all [TDHS, 13]). Of the married couples interviewed, most said that they were currently using some sort of family planning method (see fig. 6.2). These remarkably high rates of contraceptive usage by married couples of reproductive age suggest that uptake of contraceptive services is high and reinforces the claim that the Chagga are on the forefront of Tanzanian national demographic trends. The district MCH coordinator summed up her assessment of the high levels of contraceptive

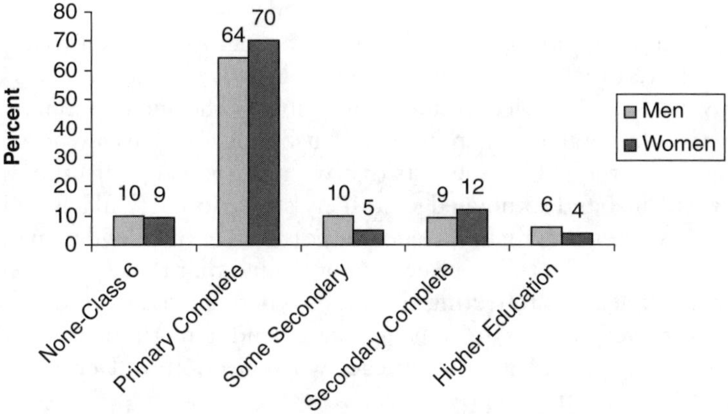

Figure 6.1 Highest Level of Education

Source: 3M Project Survey Data; Men n=246 Women n=242.

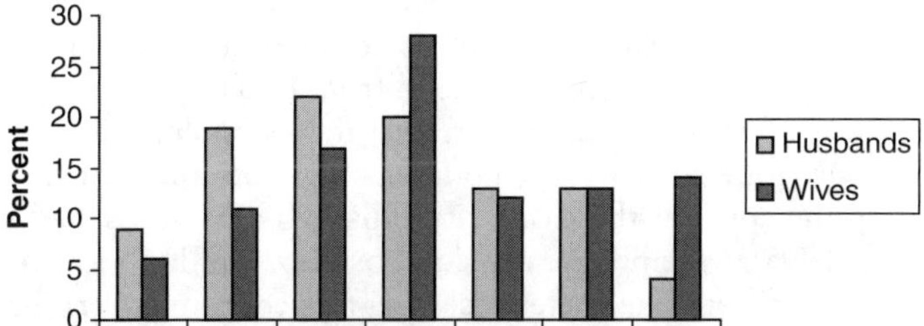

	Withdrawal	Calendar	PIlls	Injection	IUD	Sterilization	No meth
Husbands	9	19	22	20	13	13	4
Wives	6	11	17	28	12	13	14

Figure 6.2 Current Method of Family Planning

Source: 3M Project Survey Data; Men n= 254; Women n=222.

* Note that category "withdrawal" includes the other less-frequently used methods of condoms, Norplant, and abstinence.

prevalence in Kilimanjaro: "Men have already seen tough times! They agree that their wives should use family planning."

It is interesting that even though MCH clinics remain, in effect, women-only spaces, service providers emphasize that men are central to reproductive decision making and family planning. While male agreement may present the important difference between Kilimanjaro and other areas of the country, there are also wives who are choosing to use family planning, or to use modern methods, when their husbands have other ideas as we see in table 6.3. Of the methods currently used by married couples, injection is the most popular and there is a large gender gap between husbands and wives who report using the method. This suggests that women are using injection without their husband's knowledge, a likely scenario particularly in light of the reverse gender gap in reporting of the use of calendar method. In follow-up in-depth interviews, I confirmed that these gaps were at least in some cases reflecting situations where husbands told me that they were very successfully using the calendar method, while their wives were supplementing its efficacy with injections of Depo-Provera or swallowing contraceptive pills.

One illustrative example is the Mwasha family who live in a relatively affluent section of the village in a well-built, painted cement house set back from the road in a grassy garden. Mrs. Mwasha and I spoke in a sitting room furnished with a basic and rather old sofa set and wooden cabinets. The walls were decorated sparsely with a plastic clock and a large and colorful poster of Jesus, and a multicolored fuzzy brush sat on the coffee table in front of us. The family is on the lower side of affluence in local terms: for example, they have wired their house for electricity, even purchasing lights and bulbs, but could not pay the costs of the electricity bills. Mrs. Mwasha had her first child in 1995 at the private mission hospital, and her second in 1998 at the government one. After receiving advice from government project workers and the church that she should not give birth in rapid succession [*usizae haraka sana*] because life today is difficult, she began to use pills after the birth of her first child. She used them until she wanted another pregnancy and then stopped. After the second child was born, she went to the dispensary for advice because she had problems with weight loss that she attributed to the pills. Her child was three months old, and she began using Depo-Provera, but could not tolerate the bleeding so she stopped after two shots. When I interviewed her, she had been using the calendar method for a year and thought that it was a good idea. She said that she planned to use it until they want another child. After that, she said that she will probably go back to the clinic for advice, or she will go sooner if the calendar fails her.

Her husband, however, told a different story. He explained that he and his wife had discussed together the issue of childspacing and that they had used the calendar method after the birth of their first child to wait before having another one. After the second child, they used the calendar as well. He told me clearly that they had never used any other method of contraception because he had heard that they have side effects. I inquired as to where and what he had heard about side effects and he replied that when he was talking with groups of young men or elders, they told about condoms and Norplant and about their related health problems. It is interesting that both Mr. and Mrs. Mwasha agreed that they talk together and decide together on fertility issues, but there was clearly a period when she was using modern contraception without his knowledge. They both spoke at ease about their relationship and decision making.

Side effects were reported as a main concern for husbands twice as often as for wives when making decisions about choosing a method of family planning as shown in fig. 6.3 and 6.4. In interviews, husbands often expressed fear of side effects of modern methods. Husbands even voiced concern that certain methods would negatively affect their own health, as well as that of their wives. Furthermore, concern for the possibility of fertility in the future was an almost universal concern for men and women, even for those who already had many children. Six percent of husbands and twelve percent of wives responded that safety while breastfeeding was their primary concern with a method. This is particularly important in the ongoing calculus of the health of existing children and the possibility of another pregnancy. Perhaps the husbands' concern for their wives' health translates into the use of traditional, but less effective methods, as Johnson-Hanks (2002) found in Cameroon, while the wives' concern for their own health may result in using the most effective method

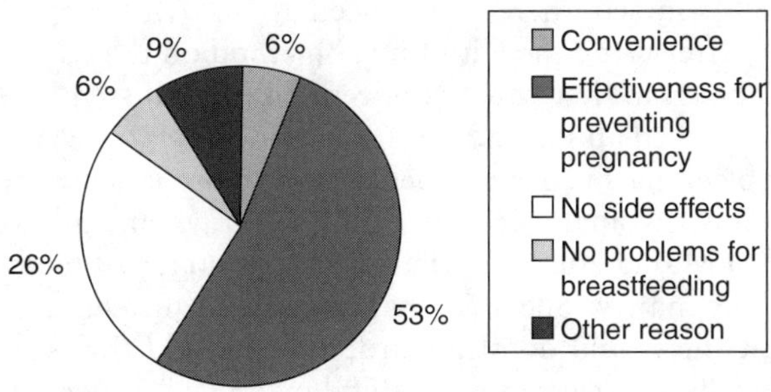

Figure 6.3 Most Important Reasons for Choosing a Particular Contraceptive Method—Husbands

Source: 3M Project Survey Data.

possible and tolerable for avoiding a mistimed pregnancy. Still, both reported "effectiveness for preventing pregnancy" as the most important consideration when choosing a method.

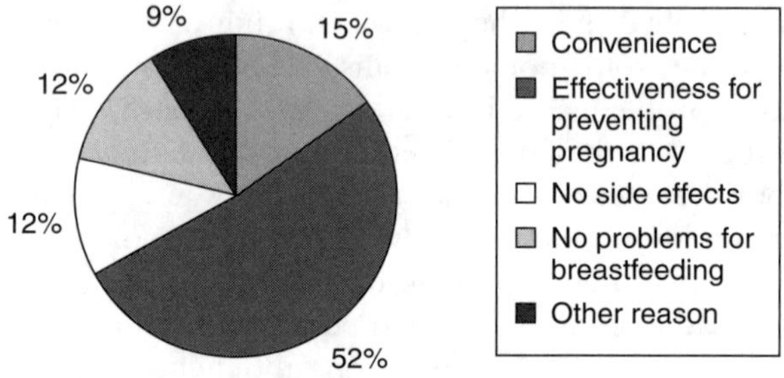

Figure 6.4 Most Important Reasons for Choosing a Particular Contraceptive Method—Wives

Source: 3M Project Survey Data.

The following narrative provides one example of the complex relationship between traditional and modern family planning choices and fertility control in the lives of rural Tanzanians. The Husseini family lives in a very basic cement house with a dirt courtyard and two small mud buildings for cooking and other work or storage. In separate interviews, they explained a bit about how decision making and family planning occurred in their household. Baba Husseini has five children to care for and would not be happy to have another one—"Five are enough!" he told me. But, he and Mama Husseini do not use contraceptives because they would be dangerous for her health—"Her reproductive organs would be hurt by the poison in that medicine; if you respect yourself there is no need to use those medicines" he explained. After using the withdrawal method on the advice of a relative to space their first three children, Mama Husseini went to the clinic and received an injection of Depo-Provera. However, because of the heavy bleeding she decided herself not to use it again, and instead went to a local woman for a drinkable mixture of traditional medicine. I asked Mama Husseini what she might do if this method fails to prevent a pregnancy. She said that she would just have the child. I asked what she would do afterward, and she said that she would go back to the clinic to get more "hospital methods." When I asked Baba Husseini about household decision making, he told me that he decides himself, and then they plan together. Then he elaborated that they would talk about things first, and then "God himself" would make the decision. Again, we see neither the calculated planning of the family by individuals promoted by the modernist, demographic discourse, nor the resignation of procreation to the will of the divine characterized by traditional ideologies. Baba Husseini, Mama Husseini, and "God himself," seemingly in that order, assess the contingencies of the Husseini household and act to try to bring a favorable outcome.

When asked to assess some of the popular statements about children in terms of their relevance to the contemporary or historical context of fertility decision making, husbands and wives gave similar responses, which are summarized in fig. 6.5. Most agreed that "children help their parents in old age" and "children give prestige" were more true in the past than in contemporary Kilimanjaro. However, nearly 70 percent agreed that "children are expensive" is more true today, and the cost of children as a factor in deciding to have a child was a common theme in interviews.

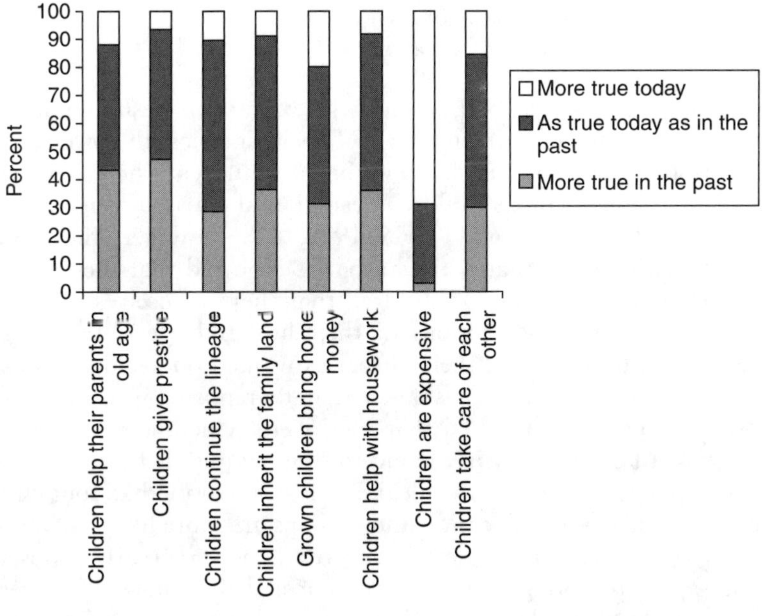

Figure 6.5 Perceptions of the Changing Role of Children in the Family Context
Source: 3M Project Survey Data.

We are reminded of Aikande's explanation that childspacing was necessary to take care of the child you already have. Another indicator that the context of reproductive decision-making in Kilimanjaro differs both from Bledsoe's Gambian case, and from other communities within Tanzania comes from the low number of children desired by respondents at the time of the interview (see fig. 6.6).

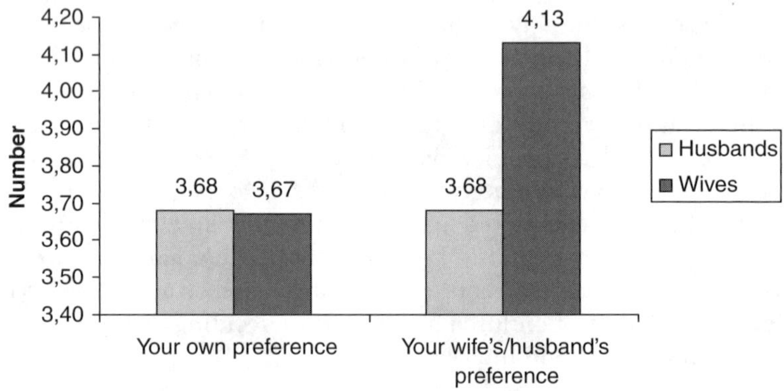

Figure 6.6 Mean Ideal Number of Children
Source: 3M Project Survey Data; Men n= 246 Women n= 242.

Husbands and wives reported almost the exact same desired number of children (means of 3.68 and 3.67). This is significantly lower than the national statistics for ideal number of children where married women had a mean of 5.7 children desired, and married men wanted a mean of 6.3 children (TRCHS 1999, 81). However, the more interesting finding is that while husbands reported that their wives wanted the same number of children that they themselves wanted, wives had different perceptions of their husbands' fertility preferences. Wives thought that their husbands wanted on average almost half a child more than the husbands actually reported wanting. One possible explanation may be that men were reluctant to admit to preferring a larger family in the face of the ubiquitous health education campaigns promoting the ideal family of no more than four children. Men have more education and perhaps are more likely to know the "right" answer, yet it is women who are more regularly exposed to messages promoting a small family norm at the clinics. However, another more plausible explanation may be that wives are assuming that their husbands are embracing nostalgic ideas of promoting the lineage with a big family while the men themselves are translating the realities of economic decline into desires for fewer children. Viewed from a more contextualized decision-making process, it would appear that both husbands and wives are giving their fertility preferences in light of their current situation, but women may be predicting their husbands' ideal goal for childbearing, not their actual one. Overall, the responses from married couples in Kilimanjaro Region describe a situation of high family planning use and low desired fertility, although the kinds of methods used to reach these goals are somewhat different according to men and women.

While this type of data should be interpreted cautiously, the shifting ideology on the cost-benefits of children as shown in fig. 6.6 is congruent with the demographic discourse being promoted through the National Family Planning Programme described earlier in the book. Situating the changing role of children within the larger framework of the capital economy—"Children are expensive" and "Grown children bring home money"—represents the more modern contextualization of the value of children. This local discourse fits comfortably within a national one of reducing family size to achieve economic development and the international one of the global population problem. Thinking demographically about one's family as understood through the local lens of childbearing may mean that any potential pregnancy is weighed against the needs of the existing children. Thus, in a context like that of Kilimanjaro where the local priorities are in harmony with the disciplining global logics of neoliberal modernity, the conditions for an auspicious pregnancy are difficult to achieve, and become more difficult with each additional child. Not surprisingly, in this area, the statistics tell us that fertility rates are declining yet the process behind each decision is not unlike that in other regions of the country.

Conclusions: A Well-Timed Pregnancy is Your Plan, an Ill-Timed One is God's Plan

Are modern contraceptives as brought into the Tanzanian health system through donor-funded interventions providing what Watkins, Rutenberg, and Wilkinson describe as "a powerful ally for women who have reached conclusions that differ from those of their husbands" (Watkins, Rutenberg, and Wilkinson 1997, 240)? Or, are modern contraceptives simply technologies of domination used by the apparatus of family planning to manifest the expectations of the global population discourse in which local Tanzanian women's voices are rarely, if ever, heard? This chapter has shown that they are clearly both. The global population discourse filters down to the level of everyday Tanzanians through the family planning clinic. In this environment, service providers, themselves Tanzanian women struggling to create a professional identity in conditions of scarce resources, find that the global population discourse's depiction of local women makes sense. Those women whose fertility has gone "out of control" need motivation, teaching or even a gentle push to embrace the modern disciplines of the body. Here, the global discourse intersects with local biases, based on levels of socioeconomic development, urbanization, and other perceptions of modernity and places local women in a context of disempowerment. Local bodies are not the same, neither as the preconfigured users for whom modern contraceptives were designed, nor as the traditional (backward) attitudes, nor as pools of unmet need for contraceptives.

This chapter has argued that family planning in Tanzania must be considered from a different perspective, one that is contextual, contingent, and related more to a regime of sporadic contraception than to a continuous calculus of informed method choice and parity-specific fertility desires. This is not meant to imply that there is no planning taking place in the Tanzanian context, quite the contrary. Women, and occasionally their partners, are using various methods of contraception to wait or to rest between pregnancies. However, sometimes these strategies fail, and if this happen, it is usually described as "God's plan." In a recent book on menstruation and menstrual regulation, Renne suggests that "to attribute a single interpretation or meaning to these acts not only overlooks the particularities of specific historical and sociocultural contexts but also discounts the advantage of ambiguity, which has empowered women in different times and different places with a certain reproductive authority" (Renne and Van de Walle 2001, xxxiii). Fertility decision making in general does not lend itself to singular interpretations, elegant models, or acontextual generalizations. In the context of increasing expectations about what it means to have a well-cared for child, education, and a modern life, parameters of planning narrow down to become nearly recognizable to Western discourses. However, issues on the "wantedness" of any pregnancy must be interpreted within the multifaceted context in which that pregnancy occurred, its outcome, and the steps taken to prevent or promote such an outcome. Planning one's family is not necessarily inconsistent with the belief that children come from God: if a pregnancy happens, it will just happen, but women are happy when they can plan.

The research from Kilimanjaro Region may provide some clues as to how the interpretations of contraception and childspacing are similar in communities with both low and high fertility, but the parameters that define when a pregnancy would be auspicious are different. In these contexts, contraceptive use is characterized by improvisation (Tilly 1999) as a means of interpreting the global population discourse into actions that make social sense. Bledsoe describes how in The Gambia, "the number of God-given fetuses a woman will bear as miscarriages, sickly infants, or children who can survive and prosper depends on her eroding bodily capacity to bear a child" (2002, 167). However, socioeconomic development smoothes this bodily trajectory. When the economic, psychological, and social costs of bearing children are laid over the physical toll in the cases of increasing levels of affluence, we see different priorities becoming relevant at any given time. Decision making is still best understood within a contingent life course, but the context in which a pregnancy becomes wanted becomes more difficult to achieve. Bodily senescence and fatigue may still provide an important motivation to rest before having another child. However, increasingly modern notions of socioeconomic need—particularly in the realm of education—taken in a context where each potential pregnancy is reckoned against the needs of the already existing children, make auspicious timing of many children difficult, if not impossible to achieve. Thus, family planning, through the use of traditional or modern methods, becomes a necessity. Kilimanjaro, on the basis of its higher levels of education and health care may provide us with an example of contingent decision making where some families are still using family planning to have more children, but far more are using it to have fewer.

Chapter Appendix on Data and Methodology

This chapter is an attempt to understand a local lens that must be read alongside other competing lenses of fertility and reproductive decision making. Samuel R. Delany reminds us of Foucault's insight that "while we sit discussing the word, power works in silence" (Delany 1994, 268), but nonetheless suggests ways for highlighting the structures of a given discourse. The method chosen for this chapter involves the critical observation of what is around us while remaining on the alert for things that contravene what we expect. This chapter documents observations of this discourse as transmitted through interviews, observations, and informal conversations with Tanzanian women and men. From over two years of fieldwork in Tanzanian communities, I have gained clarity and illumination regarding the diversity and complexity of these discourses, and a recognition of the immense investment that would be required ethnographically if one were to claim cultural fluency. Thus my attempts at translation of local lenses should be read as partial, ongoing, and open to reinterpretation, particularly from those whose experiences they are meant to represent.

To this end, this chapter draws on empirical data primarily from two field studies in Tanzania. The first involved 18 months of fieldwork in three Tanzanian regions in 1995–1996, and the second consisted of 6 months of fieldwork in Kilimanjaro region at the end of 2000. Both of these studies involved multiple methods of qualitative and quantitative data collection, primarily participant observation and interviews in the first, and a household study, follow-up interviews, and focus groups in the second. This chapter has drawn primarily on material gleaned from respondent interviews, most of which were with women, a fact to which I will return. My fieldwork was conducted in 10 service provision sites (equally distributed between urban clinics in the regional capital cities and clinics in the villages at varying distances from the cities) in Morogoro, Ruvuma, and Kilimanjaro Regions, and these data are analyzed together with quantitative national level survey data. Taken together, these three regions are representative of the diverse contexts of reproductive health care and family planning throughout contemporary Tanzania. Preliminary interpretations and findings were shared with the respondent communities during trips for dissemination and updating in 2002 and 2004.

The interviews analyzed in the first section of this chapter were conducted primarily in maternal and child health clinics with a sample of women, half of whom were using family planning at the time, and half who were not. I have summarized some background characteristics of the respondents in table 6.3. Because these were interviews and not surveys, and the sample was not purely random, this chapter avoids questions of statistical significance in analyzing responses. Responses have been coded and analyzed in order to be grouped into descriptive tables; however, they have also been analyzed through qualitative text analysis as well. Respondents attended the MCH clinic for a variety of reasons including coming for contraception, bringing a sick child or a child for immunizations, or accompanying someone else. I chose to interview clinic attendees because I wanted to be certain that these women had been exposed to the family planning message. As part of the regular procedures in all clinics, health education talks [*elimu ya afya*] are supposed to be given before service provision commences on any given morning. Many, if not most of these talks involve some pro-contraception message. I chose to interview women who were users and non-users of family planning in hopes of getting diverse perspectives. When I designed this research to sample women who were current users of modern family planning and women who were not current users, I anticipated that that the women who were not using contraceptives would provide me with an articulation of resistance. In contrast, I found little explicit resistance to family planning in general, or to the idea that women would and should plan their pregnancies.

Table 6.3 Descriptive Data for Respondents

Region		*Morogoro*	*Ruvuma*	*Kilimanjaro*	*Total*
Number of respondents		120	40	40	200
Average age of respondent	Years	28	27	30	28
Geographical origins	Same as interview site	53	49	55	52
	Other urban	13	14	0	9
	Other rural	35	38	45	39
Marital status	Currently in union	74	78	78	76
	Unmarried	12	10	20	14
	Divorced/ separated	11	8	3	7
	Widowed	3	5	0	3
Type of marriage	Polygamous	18	32	6	19
	Monogamous	82	68	94	81
Literacy	Literate in swahili	66	59	78	67
	Somewhat literate	11	10	8	10
	Illiterate	23	31	15	23

Continued

Table 6.3 Continued

Region		*Morogoro*	*Ruvuma*	*Kilimanjaro*	*Total*
Formal education	None	19	18	5	14
	Some primary	8	15	8	10
	Primary complete	68	60	65	64
	More than primary	3	3	13	6
	Secondary complete	3	5	10	6
	Higher	0	0	0	0
Reasons for stopping school	Doesn't know	3	0	0	1
	Parents' ability [*uwezo*]	40	31	53	42
	Failed exam	16	20	3	13
	Marriage	3	6	7	5
	Pregnancy	3	9	3	5
	Physical problem	3	6	3	4
	Family problem	17	6	0	7
	Didn't send girls	5	6	13	8
	Other	11	17	17	15
Woman's employment	None	23	13	3	13
	Farming/ herding	48	60	53	54
	Informal business	20	23	23	22
	Formal salaried employment	3	0	5	3
	Formal non-manuel	2	5	10	6
	Self employed	3	0	8	4
Partner's employment	None	1	3	0	1
	Farming/ herding	30	55	23	36
	Informal business	22	3	16	14
	Formal salaried employment	25	21	10	19
	Formal non-manuel	9	9	19	12
	Self employed	13	9	32	18

Continued

Table 6.3 Continued

Region		*Morogoro*	*Ruvuma*	*Kilimanjaro*	*Total*
Religion	Muslim	56	70	25	50
	Christian	18	18	50	29
	Catholic	26	13	25	21
Regularly attends	No	36	25	8	23
Church or Mosque	Yes	64	75	93	77
Transport	None	57	58	73	62
	Bicycle	35	38	15	29
	Motorcycle/ scooter	3	3	5	3
	Car	6	3	8	5

Source: Original Data.

Intermezzo 4

A Dissemination and Updating Visit to a Regional Hospital

This morning I went to the regional hospital. First, I noticed that the fancy entrance way has been closed off and seems to have given way to hawkers, so the main entrance is now on the other side next to the entrance to the wards instead of the offices. The fancy vehicle entrance had a little round-about [*kipi lefti*] of brightly painted striped blocks, implying effective control of traffic. It struck a particularly ironic note in the nineties when anyone who was rich enough to afford a vehicle would drive it to a private hospital, preferably a few hours away in the capital, instead of utilizing a public regional hospital. Nothing else seemed different than I had remembered—people trying to find a bit of shade in the shadows of the buildings' overhang, dust, a few white four-wheel drives coming and going. The main difference seemed to be a sign at the entrance with the fees posted on it. There was also a very small sign by the reception saying that they do not accept bribes [*rushwa haipokei hapa*].

I met with the district medical officer (DMO) in his office with an air conditioner. The DMO was very welcoming and we had a nice chat in Swahili with a few English phrases thrown in for technicalities. I asked first about decentralization since they had just started it in the mid-90s and I thought as a district officer, he would be happy to talk about it. Indeed, he said that they had gone far in the decentralization process and now had to focus on capacity building. He also said that there was a big difference in the amount of resources available. Before the decentralization, there were very few resources, but now they get them from the central government. Later in the discussion, he said that the resources they get are enough [*Sasa hivi, tuna*

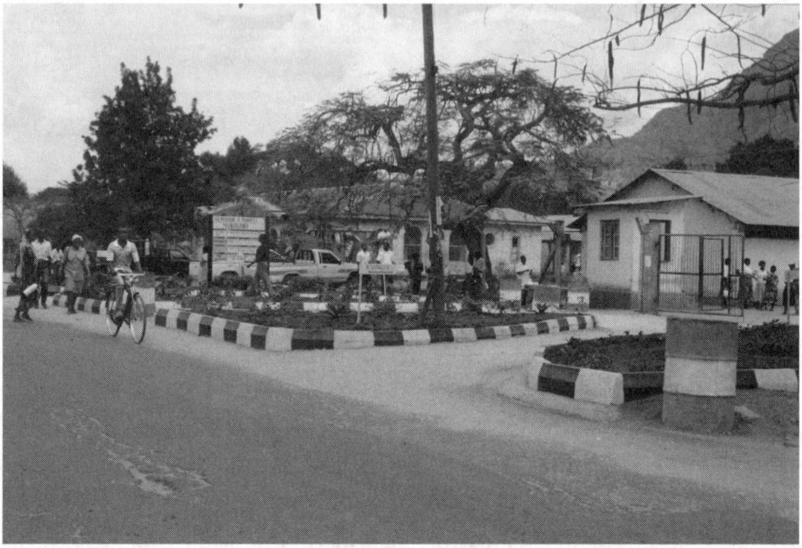

Photo 8 The Newly Painted Round-About at the Entrance of the Morogoro Regional Hospital

Source: Photograph by Lisa Ann Richey.

resources ya kutosha]. Now, they are working on the capacity of the providers.

There is a major donor project that provides much of the input. In 1995 they started with "evidence-based planning" and now they have various components. They have conducted a lot of training and built up infrastructure. They now have improved communication with fax, radio calls, internet, and even radio calls in the villages. They also have the radio and a motorbike for supervision in the villages. At first they had difficulties in how to utilize the funds—they wanted to spend $2 per capita and the district could use only 30 percent of the funds in the first year. By now they are up to $1 per capita. The planning capacity was also in need of improvement. Now they use the data from the National Health Information System to plan, but the data from the health centers are often not reliable. This particular project is finishing, but they are going on to another project to build on the things done with the earlier project. Cost-sharing has been started but only in the district and regional and consulting hospitals. This is important because people cannot expect to get health services for free. They have to contribute at least something, he said.

He lists a few other projects in the district that are run by various donors. Having not heard anything about AIDS up to this point, I asked directly about AIDS. He said they had the National Programme from the government and the World Vision would be starting a project to buy condoms, promotion, and creation of awareness. I asked about antiretroviral drugs (ARVs) and access and he said that people buy them from the capital. He expects the region, district, and consulting hospitals to get them eventually, after capacity building.

I asked him to compare 2004 with the 1990s: "Now there are even ten times more funds. Now if you go to a government hospital there are committed workers. They get enough medicine. If you go to a government hospital and there is not mismanagement, you will see that the government is doing its job. Now they examine the burden of disease and they order the medicines from the stores. Of course some workers do not order the drugs properly when they look through their stores, but it should be working and drugs should be available."

I said that I was glad to hear that things were going so well and I wondered if they had any problems now. He said the biggest problems were "health seeking behavior." I asked for clarification and he explained that "people come very late and then they are too late. If they come on time they have the drugs and staff." Why do they come late? People go first to the traditional healers. Data show that 70 percent go first to traditional healers (I clarified this number in Swahili and it was correct). The second problem was accessibility in some areas—the bad roads and flooding during the rainy season is still a big problem.

Also, referrals were still a problem from the rural health centers and clinics to the hospitals. People are afraid to travel to the hospitals that they will not have enough money and do not know how much it will cost or they do not come because the transport is difficult. Also, if there is a problem it is difficult to get the providers to refer people. I asked about integration and he said that the vertical programs have started to decrease a bit. When the government does the planning, they want integration so the donors have started to see this and have less vertical programs. Also, sustainability is an issue. Insurance and community health funds are important. You cannot get anything for free and so people must contribute. I asked if they will pay or just go more to traditional healers, he said that education is very important.

I was a bit astounded to think of how things really look exactly the same, except for his air conditioner, but seem to be so different in terms of resource availability. I decided to go to the MCH/FP clinic.

Compared to my previous work, the district was better endowed as the beneficiary of a large health intervention by donors, and the planning and procurement of supplies seemed to go more smoothly, at least as perceived from the top of the administration. The DMO's articulation of bad culture practices and weak infrastructure as the ongoing constraints to health care provision were no different than in the past. From my historical experience in the actual clinics, I wondered if they now had sufficient fuel for the motorcycles, if the staff actually ever went on the scheduled supervision visits, and why people continued to choose traditional healers, refused to follow referral advice, and worried about the cost of services.

If I had left after meeting with the DMO, I might have taken with me the idea that the dilapidated clinics, shortages of supplies that were not contraceptives, and push to get Tanzanian women to adopt permanent and long-term methods of family planning I had experienced in the fieldwork, had been transformed by a 10-fold increase in funds and efficiency. However, there is a considerable distance from the policies to the clinics and between the air-conditioned office of the district health leadership and the MCH/FP clinic a few footsteps away. Let us now consider the view from the clinic on that same morning:

The clinic was as I remember, with women and children packing the outer room and a nurse sorting cards at the reception. The family planning room had not changed except there are now cardboard boxes for every year starting in 1993 (filed together with 1994 since there are so few cards) piled on top of the chairs and broken cabinet. There were at least 30 clients for family planning whom I saw throughout my visit, and the procedures were similar, except that Mama Maria was the only provider. I remember Mama Maria as one of at least four or five others. Now, she was in a small room behind a blue cloth at the far left hand side with all the clients for family planning. When I went into the room, the examination table was covered with empty boxes of Depo-Provera and assorted discarded papers. There was hardly a chair available for a client. The walls in the clinic were covered in some of the same posters from the nineties and a couple of new ones from a different project. I was a bit surprised to see everything looking much the same, if perhaps a bit more crowded. There were two wooden doors, one signed "store" and one signed "sister."

I went into "sister" and found two nurses, one of whom I knew from when I was here before, Mama Anna. She was at a table in a room crowded with dusty Depo boxes and old papers. The table held various testing vials of something liquid (I did not ask what it was) and assorted pieces of paper and old notebooks. She was drawing lines in a notebook with a ruler (something I recall watching nurses do often).

After the usual greetings and inquires about families on both sides, Mama Anna told me that she had just finished a course in Mbeya and was now an HIV counselor who did testing, counseling, and MCT (Maternal to Child Transmission) treatment with ARVs. She had just started her work this week and was obviously a bit put off about it. Mama Anna explained that she had to get women to volunteer for testing, which took only a few minutes. Then they got the results right away, and if they were positive, they got ARV's for the unborn child. However, women were reluctant to test, she said. They were embarrassed because of "stigma" (an English word used in Swahili conversation). This is why they are now integrating HIV testing with antenatal care and family planning, so women can come to the clinic without being seen and get confidential testing.

She explained the work to me in a "professional" manner, but after I had been there a while, just sitting around, I overheard her talking to the other midwife. She said that she did not have any clients and she did not know what to do. She was complaining about staying with the family planning provider, and wondering if she should go to the antenatal part of the clinic. "Where am I going to get these clients?" She kept asking to no one in particular. She honestly did not seem to want to go anywhere and was complaining a long time about getting clients. I was unclear if she was asking the nurse to help her find clients, to test herself, or to do something else. Nonetheless, I finally asked Mama Anna if she had to get a certain number of clients. She said she had to test four women per day. Trying to lighten things up a bit, I joked that perhaps she could just snatch them off the busy road outside. She laughed and said, no, they had to be voluntary, but anyone in the clinic was fine. I asked if she had had to give anyone the news that they were HIV positive and she replied that so far, she had not, but she said it would be really difficult to do so. The other nurse Sara agreed. She said that if a pregnant woman was positive, they would give her the ARVs and advise her not to breastfeed, but if that did not work, they would advise her to breastfeed exclusively for six months and then stop abruptly. I asked if people here were accustomed to exclusive breastfeeding, or if they usually started to supplement breastfeeding early with other foods like in the rest of Tanzania. The nurses said that most people supplement early and do not breastfeed exclusively. I then asked if the nurses thought that most women would be able to manage to follow the recommended regime. Without hesitation, both nurses said "No. They won't agree to it" [*Hawakubali*].

Their project included a blurred photocopy of a questionnaire in English, which they had to fill out for each client. Mama Anna was worrying about filling in this form as well. As I was leaving, they had found two clients and were doing the test (I was unable to see how they found them, but I know Mama Anna left the family planning part of the clinic and went elsewhere). They closed the door to the room marked "sister," and I overheard someone joking and laughing about "confidential" in English, so I suppose this was the protocol they had to follow.

While they did the test, I was in the cramped room where family planning was provided, talking to Mama Maria. She said that now they had drugs and a sterilizer with steam that works. I remarked on the water I had seen dripping from the faucet, which was dry in the past, and she agreed that the piped water was an improvement. Now they have supplies, gloves, and bleach. For the last five years or so, it has not been a big problem. Now, they have more clients all the time, but staff shortages. In all sections there is usually only one person. When I asked about AIDS, she said that they do HIV counseling and include it in the regular health education lectures. I asked about the available contraceptive methods and she said they have pills, Depo-Provera, and condoms. They have not had foam or spermicide tablets now for at least three years, and still have no diaphragms or female condoms. Since October 2002, they have had no IUDs or Norplant contraceptive implants that had been highly promoted methods in the mid-1990s. Mama Maria had no idea why they no longer use these methods.

She told me that most clients use Depo-Provera injections, and then pills but now many also use condoms. They use condoms mostly to prevent STDs. When I asked about men in the clinic, she clarified that only women come, but they take the condoms too. They do a rapid test for syphilis and treat it in the clinic. Drugs are available from a donor project. Mama Maria said that they had not actually received the antiretroviral drugs PMTCT but would get them after training—it will help, she said, especially the kids. (And only for them since the mothers themselves will not be given treatment.) When I asked Mama Maria if she thought that women would manage the recommended regime for preventing vertical transmission of HIV, she said that the mothers will try it if they are able to keep the kids well, but the problem will be the formula. Where will it come from? We need a project to supply formula, she said. She had seen a flier somewhere of such a project but has not seen anything about it in the clinic yet. For other AIDS treatment, she named a doctor who has a clinic to test CD4 and get ARVs at the country's largest hospital, so people go to the capital for treatment. She did not know if it was expensive or if many people actually went. When I asked about other reproductive health services like treating infections, Mama Maria said that once a year they do a pelvic exam on clients in the adjoining room (also used today for the AIDS test mixing). People with STDs have increased a lot—I asked why this is the case if they are using condoms. She said that, of course, not everyone uses condoms, and not all the time. They use condoms at first, and then when they know their partner, they stop. If men need to treat STDs, then they must go to the doctor at the hospital for treatment.

7

Conclusion

Global discourses on population have material and symbolic effects on local politics, service provision, and reproductive decision making. The effects of such discourses can be seen in the narratives between donors and the state, between service providers and their clients, and between husbands and wives. Meanings are negotiated, deals are struck, and families are planned within a global discourse, yet everyone is local somewhere. Not surprisingly, discontent emerges at the interface of such a predetermined, static, and homogeneous solution to complex and contingent local problems.

Tanzania's National Population Policy was created through the struggle between governing bodies into modern self-regulation and many levels of local where interpretations of meaning and practicalities of practice prevail. The state, donors and lenders, and implementing organizations struggled to make meaningful policy through accommodative bargaining. Each sought to defend its own interests and the support of its constituency through polyvalent performances, such as the shifting meanings of the population problem. The international and national politics behind sensitization to the problem, foot-dragging in adoption and implementation, and the multiple discourses of the document text itself, extend both into the field of implementation in clinics, and into the future in facing the challenges of promoting reproductive health in a time of HIV/AIDS.

The Integrated Project analyzed in chapter four may provide us with a proxy for understanding the complexity of implementing reproductive health projects over time, since it was designed to integrate feminist, development, and demographic concerns. If so, the lesson would be that donor politics, gender relations, and economic needs are not necessarily compatible with a feminist vision of women's empowerment. Reproductive health will not succeed in Tanzanian villages if it is understood as merely contraceptive promotion with other interventions added on. Contraceptive technologies are quintessentially modern in their global origins and in their local meanings. The politics of category formation around contextual meanings of modern family planning reflect the national and international discourses and contingent, local hierarchies. Service providers are caught up in these modernity struggles, trying to reconcile increasing contraceptive prevalence, inadequate clinic facilities, and their own identities as modern women. In response, local women and men do, at times, accept family planning and use modern contraceptives. However, local lenses for understanding these technologies and their value emphasize planning for families. The contingency of a propitious birth is overdetermined by multiple understandings of individual women, their partners, and their social and economic situation. The meaning-making project of neoliberal modernity that shapes the global discourse on population also moulds reproductive decision

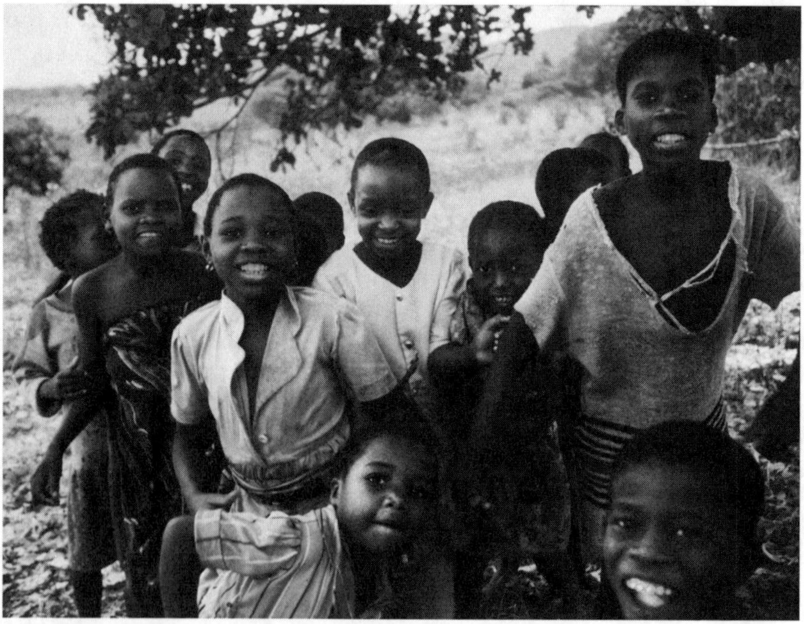

Photo 9 A Group of Children Playing on a Sunday Afternoon

Source: Photograph by Lisa Ann Richey.

making of local women and men. Bringing up your child well in the context of the realities of a "tough life" [*maisha magumu*] is an increasingly complicated affair. It is not surprising that Tanzanians are becoming increasingly savvy in planning their families.

Post-Cairo Shift: The Local Meaning of Reproductive Health after a Decade

In the decade after the Cairo Conference we have seen a dramatic shift in the meaning of reproductive health in Africa. Reproductive health and rights agendas have focused attention on important issues that had not been emphasized in population debates—who controls fertility, reproductive decision making, the ethics of contraceptive methods, and the impact of gender relations in the household, clinic, and national policy environment. Still, reproductive health is focusing more on reproduction than on health. Local lenses of family planning are instead focused quite consistently on health and the ability to reproduce and care for one's existing children.

During research dissemination visits in Dar es Salaam, Morogoro, Ruvuma, and Kilimanjaro Regions in 2000 and 2004, the local manifestations of reproductive health did not seem to reflect the global optimism. Some of the local-level changes brought about by the shift from family planning to reproductive health are easily spotted. For example, the large Norwegian-funded building at Muhimbili Hospital previously housing the Family Planning Unit has been painted with a large logo and sign that it is now the home of the Reproductive Health Unit. The Green Star logo for family planning services was launched throughout the country between 1993 and 1996: as the name implies, it is a green star with a white circle in the middle showing a healthy family surrounded by the words *Uzazi wa mpango* [family planning]. In 1998, the government began removing the words from the logo as part of the long-term repositioning to "reinforce the concept that the *Nyota ya Kijani* [green star] promotes health for the child, the mother and the whole family" (Ministry of Health 1998). Apart from such local manifestations of a discursive shift, what has become of family planning now that the population problem has been reconfigured as a lack of reproductive health services?

Visits to family planning clinics suggest similar patterns of consistency and change in the post-Cairo decade. Local clinics are still dependent on whatever project is taking place to supply inputs and training for health care. In the mid-1990s, family planning was a substantial provider. Now it is not. Some MCH service providers who were trained in family planning are now being retrained for HIV/AIDS testing and counseling. Instead of the desirable effect of integrating these important elements of reproductive health into routine provision of family planning services, the new demands of preventing maternal to child HIV transmission appear to have replaced those of family planning.

In this context, integration has come to mean one contraceptive service provider handling 30 to 40 clients per day. Having examined the daily client logs from different, popular clinics in 2004, this ratio appears to be the norm rather than the exception. The extensive "counseling for informed choice" of the mid-1990s appears to have been replaced by a more time-effective regime of simply asking the client, "what method do you want?" and occasionally "do you have any problems?" Methods available are effectively limited to condoms[1] and those that are most effective at preventing pregnancy while being least reliant on more highly trained providers, that is, injections and pills.[2] The emphasis on permanent and long-term methods—IUDs, Norplant, and sterilization—seems to have gone by the wayside.[3] Female-controlled methods such as the diaphragm or female condom have never been part of the modern family planning repertoire of services.

USAID's major push in Tanzanian family planning concluded in 1999. Between 1996 and 1999, there was a lull in government family planning activity as the focus became more logistic and the orientation moved from provision of services to planning and management issues (Chen and Guilkey 2003, 10). While contraceptive use increased at a fast pace in the beginning of the family planning program in the early 1990s, the end of the decade saw a slower rate of contraceptive uptake. Chen and Guilkey's statistical models suggest that this was because there were no meaningful improvements in the availability of contraceptives, the training of rural service providers, or increased IEC efforts at the end of the decade (Ibid.).

Without the push from large-scale donor interventions, Tanzanian women appear to be turning increasingly to innovation and self-help for contraceptives. Private practitioners of all sorts and pharmacists are becoming increasingly important providers of family planning services. Green's work in rural clinics argues that informal practitioners are preferred to attending government clinics, especially by poor people (Green 2000). Private providers allow people to evade "the extractive social relations which have come to characterise the latter" while maintaining access to the medicine itself (Ibid., 417). National surveys have documented an increasing role of pharmacies in supplying modern contraceptives to women: in 1991 only 2 percent of women listed pharmacies as a source in rural areas but by 1999 4.3 percent reported pharmacies (Chen and Guilkey 2003, 10). While these numbers are still quite small, it is easy to understand why women would avoid seeking contraceptives from clinics where they must negotiate a complex web of social relationships as described in this book, and in return they do not get any more actual health care or greater method choice.

National reproductive health programs in developing countries like Tanzania are implemented through the same structures of the old population policies. While the global discourse has shifted to emphasize feminist and development narratives, the demographic narrative remains in place locally. Yet, actual practices of family planning and reproductive decision making continue to challenge any top-down ordering logic. For example, fertility choices present an interesting quandary for some of the proponents of the global reproductive health agenda. Bledsoe elucidates the dual intentionality when "African

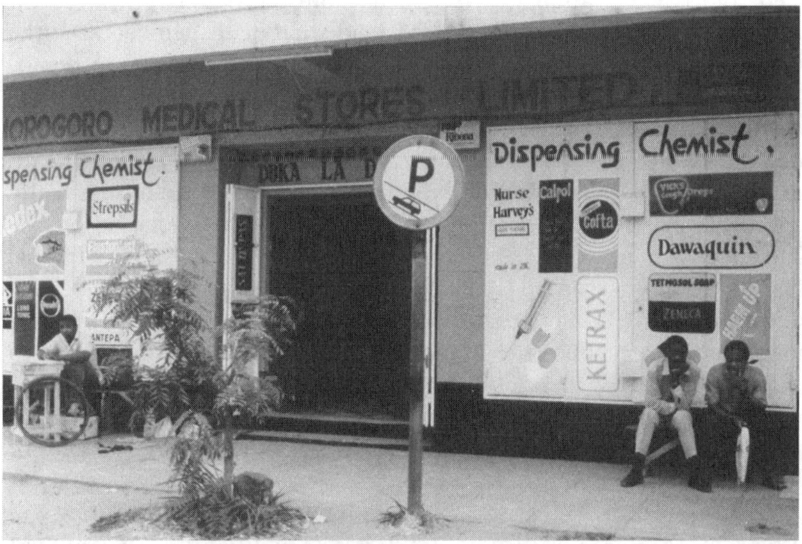

Photo 10 The Morogoro Medical Stores, a Popular Place for Purchasing Drugs and Supplies Near to the Regional Hospital

Source: Photograph by Lisa Ann Richey.

women are adopting contraceptives for the public reasons we urged them to, yet their purposes—and quite possibly their achieved empirical outcomes—contravene entirely our private intentions" (Bledsoe 2002, 328). It would be an unfair characterization to generalize motivations of the many diverse interests from all parts of the geopolitical spectrum that supported the Cairo shift from fertility control to reproductive health. However, to the extent that the interests that were most vocal in supporting previous population control ideologies have warmed to the Cairo vision as described in chapter one, it has been on the basis of arguments like that of unmet need[4] that link giving women more options and more choices, with the likelihood that they will choose to have fewer children.

Whither the Problem of Overpopulation in the Global Discourse?

Global Demographic Convergence

The contemporary demographic narrative presents a more nuanced version of the overpopulation problem when relating to Africa. We find some of the language brought in from reproductive health, but there is still little health focus and inadequate engagement with the impact of AIDS. The challenges that African data present to demographic theories are usually not used to direct a rethinking of the theories in light of their inability to explain in Africa, but are cordoned off into categories of outliers, commonly known as "African exceptionalism." For example, whether or not overpopulation is really a central problem for economic development often focuses on the capacity to meet food needs, the subject of debates since Malthus (1914)[5] and Boserup's (1970) response. Contemporary analysis of agrarian change and population growth supports the view that societies are able to produce the right institutional, economic responses to shifting demographics. However, Cuffaro (1997) argues that this optimism may not be justified in the context of very fast population growth and/or already high population densities, or in contexts of high inequality, inappropriate policies, or drought. From Cuffaro's description of the exceptions, we can expect that most societies will alter their responses to demographic change in order to thrive, but not Africa.

The notion of a *global demographic convergence* is foundational to demographic transition theory.[6] In layperson's terms, demographic transition theory says that countries will progress over time from situations characterized by high mortality and high fertility to those characterized by low mortality and fertility. Today, cross-national demographic data is sometimes used to declare an end to the population explosion.[7] Wilson (2001) describes a "global demographic change of unprecedented magnitude," with most countries moving closer and closer together in terms of their fertility and mortality rates—becoming "demographically modern." After describing the global convergence of fertility rates with terms like "overwhelming," "substantial" in a "world that has been transformed" (Ibid., 165, 166), Wilson makes a note of African exceptionalism:

> Although comprising less than a quarter of the world's population, the remaining high-fertility regions will, in any of the UN's future scenarios, provide the *majority of the population growth* expected for the next 50 years. It is not surprising, therefore, that *addressing the reproductive health needs* of these segments of the world's population remains of the highest priority for international population policy (Ibid., 166, emphasis added).

While the rest of the world is no longer a population problem, Africa is clearly presented as being different. Here we see the dynamics of pre-Cairo population control. Though they are numerically few, the Africans are responsible for a continuing population problem and therefore, they are to be the focus of *international* population policy. Placing responsibility for governing African populations in the international, as opposed to the national or local realm suggests that African population problems are primarily international problems—they exceed national boundaries—not problems of primary concern for national development or individual or family well-being. Also, the approach for dealing with these problems, "addressing the reproductive health needs" of Africans, is predicated upon the belief that their "needs" are contraceptive. Thus, meeting these needs would bring down population growth. Therefore, we can reconcile the demographic truth that the rates of population growth are indeed declining, with a vision of overpopulation as a major development obstacle in Africa. As one author has described, "there are two parallel worlds: one world in which fertility is low and declining as economic development advances, and another world where fertility remains high and where much of the population is mired in poverty" (Ashford 2001, 41).[8]

Cohen's (1998) analysis of national surveys on fertility transition in sub-Saharan Africa challenges the popular perception that the continent is demographically "stuck" in regimes of high fertility. He shows that a widespread decline in fertility is taking place, virtually across the board, and that there has been almost no survey in the last 10 years that indicates that fertility is increasing and very few suggesting it to be stationary (p. 1445). "Instead, virtually all recent surveys point to rising age at marriage, rising contraceptive use, and declining fertility, particularly amongst certain well-defined subgroups" (Ibid.). Cohen's work attributes much of this success to family planning, and he notes the "large body of evidence [that] points to the need to increase the level of family planning services in Africa" (Ibid., 1445). He concludes his description of declining African fertility with the point that "it is important to note that despite the fact that fertility is declining, the population of sub-Saharan Africa is still expected to double within the next 22–23 years" (Ibid.). Thus, the demographic momentum (Keyfitz 1977) of the population structure will continue to contribute to a population problem even when individuals change their fertility behavior. In such a meticulous examination of the demographic literature on fertility and its determinants in Africa, Cohen makes not a single mention of AIDS.[9]

The impact of the AIDS pandemic on all aspects of development policymaking will become even more pronounced as the empirical results documenting the disease are forthcoming (such as Heuveline 2003). Scholarship has shown that HIV itself has a direct impact on reducing fertility (Carpenter, Nakiyingi, et al. 1997; du Lou, Msellati, et al. 1999; Gregson, Zaba, et al. 1999 cited in Baylies and Bujra 2000). One of the first articles in a population journal to document the impact of HIV/AIDS on mortality shows that Zimbabwe experienced a massive rise in adult mortality risks from the mid-1980s to the mid-1990s (Feeney 2001). The piece concludes that "there is essentially no doubt that these increases in adult mortality risks are due to HIV/AIDS. Given the timing, age pattern, and magnitude of the changes, no competing explanation is remotely credible" (Ibid., 779). Anecdotal evidence from MCH clinics in Tanzania in 2000 and 2004 confirms increasing levels of maternal mortality and stillborn infants, which service providers attribute to AIDS. A recent literature review suggest that AIDS will have a significant detrimental impact on achievement of the Millennium Development Goals in highly affected countries (Hecht et al. 2006). As the impact of HIV/AIDS on African mortality is more accurately documented, these radical demographic facts must be taken seriously in any conceptualization of what any population policy should do in Africa.

(Dis)Integration of Reproductive Health Promotion and HIV/AIDS Interventions

Whether reproductive health will have a considerable impact on mainstream demography or on population policy practice is still unsubstantiated.[10] Within the population discourse, some old-guard demographers are still trying to wrestle the agenda back from the women's health advocates,[11] but these two sides struggle within what is essentially not a health or development discourse, but a family planning one. The critical foundation of reproductive rights as human rights has been largely unimplemented and grossly underfunded in spite of international rhetorical commitments (see Chesler 2006). The drive to integrate HIV/AIDS prevention and treatment into family planning as part of reproductive health has been mired in controversy, as the contemporary struggles of Mama Anna described in the previous intermezzo suggest. A population discourse dominated by concern for controlling fertility by women, couples, or governments precludes adequate incorporation of the challenges that AIDS brings to healthcare policy and development policies.

Contemporary family planning services must be provided under the rubric of reproductive health, including HIV/AIDS, and within a context of health care decentralization (see Askew and Berer 2003). My clinic level observations in 2000 and 2004 are consistent with other types of evaluation done in Tanzania. For example, a recent assessment was conducted at central, regional, and district levels examining the success of integrating comprehensive reproductive health services into a well-functioning health system. This study described a situation where planning and management were not synchronized either horizontally or vertically and implementation of integrated reproductive health services had been stalled, even after more than 15 years of health sector reform and a decade after Cairo (Oliff et al. 2003). However, interventions continue to be donor-driven as they were under the National Population Policy described earlier in the book. Oliff et al. point out: "The influence of donors, whose control over resources can distort or impede policy implementation, has been an obstacle to integrating reproductive health services, notably to incorporating HIV and sexually transmitted infection (STI) control into comprehensive reproductive health programmes" (Ibid., 38). While this book has demonstrated that international to local negotiations involve far more than simply money dictating policy, the priorities of donors and the structures of power that support them must be taken seriously if any meaningful improvements are to be seen in reproductive health.

HIV/AIDS threatens improvements in reproductive health by absorbing the funding and personnel so necessary to support the breadth of interventions required, and by threatening the very lives of reproductive women and men. In the push toward multisectoral responses to the HIV/AIDS epidemic, basic health care provision has failed to become sufficiently integrated as we saw in the snapshot from the MCH clinic. We can anticipate resistance from local service providers to the introduction of activities associated with HIV/AIDS that they may fear threatens their hard-earned identity as modern professionals as described in chapter six. HIV/AIDS is still associated with "stigma," immorality, and deviance and these providers have been working hard to push communities to accept their work in family planning as an important part of caring for the health of children and their mothers. A global population discourse dominated by concern for controlling fertility by women, couples, or governments precludes adequate incorporation of the challenges that AIDS brings to healthcare policy and development policies. Reproductive health in many African communities might be best understood as remaining healthy enough to reproduce.

Changing the Value of Children: Discipline and Domesticity

This book has argued that the family planning interventions seen in Tanzanian clinics are linked to a global population discourse. This discourse is made up of demographic, development and feminist narratives, all of which embrace a neoliberal vision of modern family planning. The resultant modern identity has been embraced by many Tanzanians, from service providers themselves to rural couples with hopeful visions for their children. Donors, policymakers, clinic service providers, and family planners are all engaged in performing the scripts of modernity (see Allen 2004 and Tesfaye 2003). As chapter five demonstrates, the identity artifacts of the family planning apparatus, from the modern contraceptives to the language of the posters performs a certain version of neoliberal modernity. Yet, as chapter six shows, this modernity is constantly being performed in translation.

Family planning has been demonstrated as part of the reproductive economy (Peterson 2002), where men and women negotiate their fertility desires together, often on the basis of familial, community, and cultural expectations, and then women assume the responsibility for carrying out the contraceptive tasks required by such choices. Family planning is also embedded within the productive economy both in the obviously skewed international political economy of aid, trade, and debt at the level of nation state, and in decision making around the timing of pregnancy in light of a woman and her family's resources. Finally, family planning sits within the virtual economy as a way of introducing market logic into private life. To respect oneself [*kujiheshima*] requires bodily discipline. Tanzanian policymakers were taught to think demographically in terms of population versus development, and women were instructed to use family planning to care for their children, families, and the nation. Planning one's family in the ways promoted by the global population discourse—neither having children too soon, too late, or too many—is one of the most prominent signs of one's modernity.

The disciplining of familial, social, and cultural differentiation into something "readable" within neoliberal ideology in ways analogous to the German foresters' "normal tree" as described in the introduction is not surprisingly an unattainable task in the real context of Tanzanian family planning. Yet, this is exactly the highly political, normative project of the global population discourse and its implementation arm, the family planning apparatus.

In an aptly titled chapter, "Expectations of Domesticity," Ferguson (1999) describes how definitions of the family, the household, and the good life are intertwined with highly modernist schemas into which African familial life can rarely be fitted. However, "like streamlined refrigerators, 'modern families' might be attractive for reasons that had little to do with matters of function narrowly conceived . . . [they] implied both a dream and a promise: that up-to-date modern ways belonged at home" (Ibid., 169).

Family planning comes as an agent of modernity—promising that the difficult societal costs of fertility control (side effects, gender relations, lineage and cultural values) will have significant payoffs in the material realm of increased development (education, good food, better health). Parents are lured with the promise that having fewer children will not leave them more vulnerable (fewer children to bring home remittances, fewer to look after the tasks of farm, lineage obligations, elder and child care)—that these "quality" children who are the recipients of larger investments, will actually provide greater payoffs for their families in the end. The "value" of children is shifted and a higher-risk strategy for the family is taken (which may still be a lower-risk strategy for the mother in terms of maternal health and the risk of each pregnancy).[12] The push to shift child-valuing strategies comes at the same time as promises of a recovering economy, with a new liberalized and competitive market where individuals who are most competent and effective will receive higher rewards for their abilities than in the past socialist system. In such an economic climate, it is reasonable for parents to think of investing in fewer children whom they can endow with better preparation and skills for competing in the private sphere, in hopes that they will in return, respond to the needs of the family when they have the means to do so. Yet, now the HIV/AIDS pandemic threatens to reconfigure the context of such choices in ways that makes previous thinking on investing in quality and valued children irrelevant, as these well-planned families crash against the crucible of a disease that is impossible to cure and too expensive to treat.

Reintegrating Culture into Material Analyses

The analysis of this book argues that to understand how and why global projects are countered by local failures (or limited successes, as we might claim of family planning), we must look to the mechanisms that mediate the interface between the standardizing truths and the complexity of lived social existence. This does not lend itself to parsimonious models of reproductive behavior. In fact, it requires that analysis consider that every moment of "data" is actually reflecting a conglomeration of meaning, facts, and levels of understanding, and that both the researcher and the researched are improvising to suit the circumstances. The Tanzanian case suggests that fertility choices, service provision, and policy decisions are embedded in a culture and politics that reflect both global and local discourses. Thus, the previous chapters attempt to reintegrate culture, as understood by the meanings that people give in the ways that they speak and the context or contingency of their actions, and materialist analyses.

To understand the intersections between top-down and bottom-up expressions of power, this book has indicated places where mechanisms are still functioning between the global population discourse and Tanzanian reproductive social realities. However, we can expect these mechanisms to fail or to "generate destructive incompatibility" in the following cases: "where little previous communication between local and large scale has occurred, where local connections and resources have diminished, where time horizons are shortened, and where authorities are responding to serious struggles with their own peers or predators rather than to relations with their subordinates" (Tilly 1999, 350). The crisis of HIV/AIDS together with the broad agenda and vastness of reproductive health is likely to create exacerbate such conditions in countries like Tanzania.

Family planning is not ordering one's fertility in accordance with a Platonic abstract of the "ideal number of children" but a process of ongoing decision making, based on life's contingencies. Family planning, or contracepting represents a series of material practices. Women use actual devices or engage in behaviors that result in physical, embodied consequences—they have pregnancies or not, they have side effects or not. Family planning practices also have a level of meaning that is symbolic—defining oneself as a particular type of person. The outcome of planning one's family, usually articulated as not having births too close together, but also in some cases, as not having more children than you could care for, was important in women's self-understanding of who was modern and who was not. The use of modern contraceptives, like their traditional counterparts were most often described by women as a means for preventing pregnancies that came too soon—this imperative was commonly articulated in terms of the health and well-being of the woman's other children. The global population discourse provides a neoliberal valuation of life quality as local institutions, including families, increasingly yield to the ownership society.

Focusing the message of family planning on the needs of children enables women who want to use contraceptives to appropriate this discourse of "the good mother" to legitimate their decision. This is a strong counterargument to male fears that contraceptive use will make women promiscuous. Also, linking the health of mothers to the health of their children, and the emphasis on family planning as important for maternal health, provide women with another strategy to justify choices to use contraception. In Tanzania, fertility is negotiated within a context shaped by childbearing as an integral part of gender identity, the potential threat posed by untimely pregnancy for both the mother and the existing children, and the modern notion of caring properly for one's family. Family planning is promoted and interpreted as a part of responsible parenthood, not as an alternative to it.

Notes

Chapter 1 Introduction

1. I have chosen the term "Third World" for its explicitly political meaning in the context of what is normally a discourse smoothed by globalization rhetoric. Johnson-Odim aptly defines the "Third World" as "underdeveloped/overexploited geopolitical entities, i.e. countries, regions, and even continents; and to refer to oppressed nationalities from these world areas who are now resident in 'developed' First World countries" (1991, 314).
2. As described by Peterson, this involves "cultural norms, demographic dynamics, reproductive technologies, and disciplinary regimes in regard to sex/affective relations. It also includes the meaning and valorization of erotic desires and sexual expressions (e.g. globalized media representations, sex tourism), agency and identities in relation to biological reproduction (e.g. 'bride markets,' international adoptions), conditions of health, choice and technologies of reproduction (e.g. expensive fertilization clinics for some, forced sterilization for 'others'), and the spatial and temporal constitution of social relations ('families,' support groups, communities) that enable parenting/inter-generational reproduction" (Peterson 2002, 10).
3. Tanzania has been termed a "post-conditionality" regime, where implementing structural adjustment measures is no longer a political issue and thus, donors use the disbursement of funds to promote further changes rather than to threaten withdrawal if a country does not live up to the conditionalities (Harrison 2001, 659). In this state of postconditionality, there is a mutual dependence between donors and the state, as the donors identify good reformers and then are anxious to see further success to justify their past policies and selection of good states for interventions.
4. The concept of bio-power has been used to examine the link between state planning and population management in India by Chatterjee and Riley 2001 and also adopted by numerous scholars who study the body, see for example Lock and Scheper-Hughes (1996).
5. Despite a new emphasis on male involvement in the post-Cairo discourse, the global population discourse still conceptualizes the problem and its solution in feminine terms.

6. The term "eugenics" was coined in 1883 by Francis Galton, a cousin of Charles Darwin, in his work *Inheritance of Faculties* that suggested that the moral attributes of a population would be improved through selective breeding in favor of increased genetic representation of those persons possessing more "natural ability" and "civic worth" (Ross 1998).
7. In 2004/2005 a new Demographic and Health Survey (DHS) was done in Tanzania, returning to the pre-Cairo language of the historical DHS. One comparable survey was published in 2000 and titled the "Reproductive and Child Health Survey." The DHS has been conducted in over 75 countries with the overall goals of providing universal, comparative measures of standard social and demographic behavior" (see Riley and McCarthy 2003). Data from these surveys are considered the "gold standard" for contemporary demographers. These are based on a political and cultural history of large-scale surveys in America that date back to the Indianapolis Fertility Study in the late 1930s (Whelpton and Kiser 1946–58). The World Fertility Survey of the 1970s and its successor the DHS are "the quintessential tools for a positivist, modernist social science like demography" (Riley and McCarthy 2003, 53). There is no need to reiterate the general critique of these surveys, their often-unacknowledged limitations, and their use for political ends (see Kirk 1996, Riedmann 1993, Szreter 1993, Watkins 1993, Cleland and Scott 1987, Hodgson 1983) but we will return to them in the specific case of Tanzania.
8. See also Abernethy (1993), Reid and Lyon (1972).
9. For a detailed history of the link between reproductive health and sexual rights with women's rights as human rights in the international arena, see Chesler (2005).
10. Hodgson and Watkins (1997) emphasize that while many actors, including those from the South, participated in the Cairo process, American neo-Malthusians and feminists had the greatest impact in determining the present cast of international population policy, and the United States remains responsible for funding much of its implementation.
11. Chatterjee and Riley (2001) have elucidated a similar argument in the case of India.
12. For the history of demography as a social and policy science, see Hodgson (1983, 1988); McNicoll (1992); Notestein (1982); Ramsden (2002) and Szreter (1993).
13. Presser diplomatically sums up this point: "Although many demographers view themselves as removed from the political scene, the fact that they rely so heavily on secondary sources for data—and on large data bases that require substantial funding—means that the boundaries and central concerns of the field are often defined by these data sources and the key players who are responsible for making them available" (Presser 2000).
14. Helzner and Shepard (1997) argue that feminists working in large population institutions can succeed in bringing about incremental change.

Chapter 2 Strategic Ambiguity: The Historical Context of the Tanzanian National Population Policy

1. Interview 95GD01b, August 13, 1995.
2. Censuses have been conducted in independent Tanzania in 1967, 1978, 1988, and 2002.
3. Interview 95ND01, August 28, 1995.
4. For a discussion of Tanzanian demographic change under colonialism see Turshen 1987.
5. Interview 95GD02, September 12, 1995.
6. "To a large extent this reluctance seems to be based on an erroneous perception of population as being solely concerned with fertility regulation" (United Nations Population Fund 1979, 21).
7. Interview 95ND01, August 25, 1995.
8. The Bank traces projects supporting population activities back as far as 1970 loans to Jamaica for family planning.
9. Interview 95DD01, August 30, 1995.
10. Interview 95GD01b, August 13, 1995.
11. Interview 95GD01b, August 13, 1995.
12. Tanzania reported to the ECA: "For the next decade, the Government has accorded priority to the following programmes for which international assistance and co-operation will be needed: (a) basic data collection and processing, (b) population dynamics including analysis and training in demographic research, (c) population communication and education. Second priority is given to the formulation, implementation and evaluation of population policies and programmes, family planning programmes and population redistribution programmes" (ECA Population Division 1982, 59).
13. Data are from the National Population Policies 2001 database available at http://www.un.org/esa/population/publications/npp2001/NPPdownload.htm accessed on September 10, 2007.
14. If women use family planning, their health will improve, and thus they and their children will be more productive and present less of a strain on the national health system. "It is for the interest of the parents and children to have a small family for it is easier when one has few children to deal with poverty, provide education to the children and provide the amenities of life, maintain physical and mental health for the parents and children" (Urrio 1984, 3).
15. The cover letter to this report clarifies the intended audience stating that the original proceedings were all in Kiswahili and were translated by "the authorities" "for the benefit of the donor community" (Goppel 1987).
16. In 1986 the PPU was established as a project in the then Ministry of Finance and Planning with the financial and technical assistance of UNFPA and the ILO. The PPU was both a project and a Section of the Human Resources

Planning Department in the President's Office (Okunnu 1992, Appendix H.5, 1). The PPU is responsible for coordinating the activities of the NPP, including Population IEC, population and development activities, publications, mass media, seminars, and workshops for policymakers at the national, regional, and district levels (United Republic of Tanzania 1994, 16).

17. The committee included representatives from the Institute for Development Studies, the Demographic and Training Unit and the Department of Economics, University of Dar es Salaam (UDSM); Sokoine University of Agriculture; Umoja Wa Wanawake Tanzania (UWT); Ministries of Education, Health, Agriculture, Foreign Affairs, Environment, Justice, the Environment Management Council; and the FPU. NGOs involved in drafting the policy included UMATI, the Christian Council of Tanzania (CCT), the Tanzanian Episcopal Conference, and The National Muslim Council of Tanzania (BAKWATA).
18. Interview 95ND01, August 25, 1995.
19. The targets were: 1) to reduce the proportion of women marrying before age 20 by 50 percent between 1988 and 2000; 2) to raise the minimum age at marriage for females (age 20) and males (age 25); 3) to increase the contraceptive prevalence rate to 30 by 2000; 4) to achieve an average birth spacing of at least two years by 2000; 5) by the year 2000 direct a significant proportion of the FP services and family life education (FLE) efforts to all adult males; 6) to reduce the total fertility rate from 7 to 5 or less by 2000; 7) to reduce the infant mortality rate to 90 per thousand live births or less by 2000; 8) to moderate the rate of rural-urban migration; 9) improve the status of women (derived from pp. 14–15, para. 56) (Overseas Development Administration 1991, 34, 35).
20. The informant elaborated that this unacceptability was on the grounds that some families already had four children and would thus be left out of the policy, and a four-child target would be unfair to men in polygamous marriages. Interview 95ND01, August 25, 1995.
21. CCM, with financial assistance from UNFPA, organized seminars on "Population Policy Proposal for Regional, District, Divisional and Ward Leaders of seven regions" (Mwanza and Dar es Salaam on the mainland, and all five regions of Zanzibar). These three-day seminars took place between September and December 1991 (Okunnu 1992, Appendix H.3, 2).
22. Interview 95GD01a, September 13, 1995.
23. These seminars were held by the then Department of Economic Affairs of the CCM, and $135,631 of UNFPA funding supported seminars during a nine month period. (United Nations Population Fund 1994c, 35).
24. This political balancing act seems to be common practice. Ekanem's assessment of population policies in African countries emphasizes that the process is usually a tedious one. For example, in Liberia, eight task forces prepared drafts that were then synthesized by a ninth task force before becoming a policy (Ekanem 1988, 12).
25. Interview 95ND01, August 25, 1995.
26. Interview 95ND01, August 25, 1995.
27. The policy begins: "As mentioned earlier in the second paragraph of the first chapter, annual population growth in Tanzania is rapid and *the rate has been increasing* in the past forty years" (emphasis added) (United Republic

of Tanzania 1992, 11). However, the paragraph referred to actually gives data showing that the population growth rate did indeed increase between the 1950s and 1978, but *decreased* after this point.

28. The policy states that despite a decreasing average growth rate, there are significant differences among regions, with some growing even more slowly than they did in the 1950s and others growing much faster than before. This is not noteworthy, until we read on to the next paragraph. It states: "A further analysis of the 1978 census data reveals even a more significant but negative relationship between regional fertility levels and the corresponding proportions of urban population. This analysis also indicates that rural-urban migration is a more important determinant of urban growth in the country than natural increase" (United Republic of Tanzania 1992, 2). In other words, as urbanization increases, fertility levels decrease and for these urban areas, growth is caused by people migrating into these areas, not by women having more children. If we analyze the information from the preceding paragraph with this material in mind, we see that the national policy document's comparison of regional differentials from the examples of Mtwara and Dar es Salaam suggests the following: in areas where growth rates are particularly high, the high growth is more likely to be caused by higher migration levels, not higher fertility levels. In fact, these more urbanized areas are likely to have lower fertility levels than other areas. Ironically, if more people are moving to urban areas and then taking on the lower fertility desires associated with those areas, we may see urbanization itself as leading to lower overall fertility rates—pitting one aspect of the population policy against another.
29. The sectors addressed are: Integrated MCH/FP programs; IEC; women in development; children, youths, elderly and the disabled; agriculture, food and nutrition; environment and rural development; and training, statistics and research.

Intermezzo I An Interview at the Ministry of Health

1. AVSC at this time, stood for the "Association for Voluntary Surgical Contraception." It shifted to the "Association for Voluntary Safe Contraception" by the time I finished the first field stint, and, since March of 2002 it is called "Engender Health."

Chapter 3 Population Policy Implementation and Family Planning

1. The UNFPA mid-term review documents: "As noted earlier, inadequate accommodation is a serious constraint to the effectiveness of the PPU and hence to the effective implementation of the NPP…the lack of office space has been a long standing issue and has been recognized by the donors as a problem. In fact, funding for renovation has been made available by the

World Bank and would have been available from UNFPA upon request. Action has been lacking from government" (United Nations Population Fund 1994c, 37).

2. It may be the case that the Tanzanian government is simply being strategic by putting its money into areas where donors are less readily available, given that external funds for population issues are readily available.
3. Interview 95ND02, December 12, 1997.
4. Interview 95ND02, December 12, 1997.
5. Interview 95DD02, December 12, 1995.
6. As early as 1988, the RAPID model developed by the Futures Group was being used by more than 20 African countries. Ekanem describes the blueprint for RAPID intervention: "presentations are offered to national leaders for consideration at national conferences on population and development; the national experts are then encouraged to perform comparable research. The presentations normally cover the events that led to the government's conviction to take action on the country's population growth rate; the specific steps taken; the substance of the policy measures; and, subsequent results (both intended and unintended)" (Ekanem 1988, 12).
7. Interview 95GD01b, August 13, 1995.
8. *Kangas* are large scarves worn in pairs by almost all Tanzanian women. They usually have metaphorical messages that may be used as a means of political or personal conversation, ranging from admonishing a nosy neighbor, to supporting a political party or professing one's faith in God.
9. This example comes from Ferguson (1994, 55) who uses it to illustrate a similar movement in the "development" discourse.
10. Barrett and Tsui (1999) use a time-series regression and time-varying covariates on a sample of 114 Third World countries covering the period from 1973–1992.
11. For the case of Tanzania, Barrett and Tsui's data show USAID contributed $4,444,000 in 1992 and climbing to $6,709,000 in 1993, and $7,841,000 in 1994. Email communication with Deborah Barrett.
12. I was reminded of the ongoing governmental ambivalence during an implementation workshop. When handing out an early description of my research that included the statement: "After five years of negotiations and revisions, the National Population Policy (NPP) was adopted with the National Family Planning Programme (NFPP) as its implementing arm," a member of the Planning Commission took me aside and swiftly informed me: "The National Population Policy is more than just family planning." He also said emphatically that he had been trying to tell USAID the same thing.
13. Interview 95ND01, August 25, 1995.
14. Pragmatically, restricting injections to doctors' provision effectively places it out of the reach of most Tanzanians, given that trained doctors are in extremely short supply and usually working in the capital or major regional cities.
15. Interview 95NO11, January 29, 1996.
16. The strategies adopted under the National Health Policy were: 1) to formulate and implement promotive and preventive health programs; 2) to build

health centers (to serve 50,000 people) and dispensaries (to serve 10,000 people); 3) to train adequate mid-level health workers (medical assistants, rural medical aids, MCH Aids, health assistants, and nurses) (United Republic of Tanzania, Ministry of Health and Social Welfare 1989, 7).

17. Interview 95NO11, January 29, 1996.
18. While he was not mentioned by name, one of the most outspoken critics of the population control agenda was one of Tanzania's first trained demographers and the former head of the Demographic and Training Unit at the University of Dar es Salaam. In an interview, he explained that during his participation in workshops to develop a population policy, he emphasized that "the decline of fertility should take a long time" (personal interview, August 28, 1995). However, he was in the minority and his point did not change the content of the policy, although, he said that "people were sympathetic to it." One government informant said that the demographer's ideas "hurt his credibility among the donors who accused him wrongly of influencing the government negatively" (interview 95GD01a, September 13, 1995). The government official explained the conflict between the donors and the demographer: "When he was the head of the DTU, at one stage UNFPA held up resources to the DTU until he was removed as head. The university was just stubborn enough to refuse until his time was up...the UNFPA used all sorts of excuses to delay funds, insisting on moving people who they feel aren't promoting the project" (interview 95GD01a, September 13, 1995).
19. A memo from the programme officer of the Africa Division of UNFPA concerning UNFPA's Third Country Program's Mid-Term Review follows with an explanation of how UNFPA knew that the project objectives for the MCH/FP project were unrealistic: "We, however, *were so proud* that the Government itself had formulated this project; we realized that often in such first instances the formulators are overly optimistic; plus *we did not want to dampen the enthusiasm* of the Government—so we *allowed* these overly ambitious objectives to remain" (emphasis added) (United Nations Population Fund 1994c, annex E).
20. UNFPA conducted an evaluation showing that the proportion of MCH clinics providing child-spacing services rose from 37 percent in 1982 to 80 percent in 1987 (United Republic of Tanzania, Ministry of Health and Social Welfare 1989, 4). This is a remarkable increase of 43 percent during a 5-year period. However, the number of trained family planning service providers does not measure up to these levels. In 1987, 32 out of 150 Public Health nurses (21 percent) and 800 out of 3,000 MCH Aides (27 percent) had been trained in family planning (Ibid.) We have indications of less service provision from the January 1989 NFPP Plan of Operations, which states: "Currently about 2,000 health units out of 3,056 provide family planning services" (Ibid., 10). This is only 65 percent compared to claims of 80 percent coverage in 1987. The same report estimates that discontinuation rates outside the major cities and towns may be as high as 70–80 percent, although no data are cited for this figure.
21. In mid-1989, USAID offered to contribute \$19 or \$20 million for the program, which, according to a UNFPA document, "took everyone by surprise"

(United Nations Population Fund 1994c, annex E). At this point, the questions of institutional capacities and human resources to support such a large project had to be reconsidered. Until this time, UMATI had still been spearheading family planning in the country. Also, the director of the UNFPA family planning project became the de facto director of the USAID program, effectively consolidating the leadership of the donor contingent. Finally, "after numerous major meetings, especially with the very large contingents of USAID personnel and consultants, organizational responsibilities for family planning were redistributed" (United Nations Population Fund 1994c, annex E).

22. On the ground, it is difficult to distinguish which activities were government and which were NGO, or who was part of the government hierarchy and who was part of the donor chain of command. For example, when I asked the government research officer for access to the library at the FPU, I was told that I needed permission from USAID.
23. Interview 95DD04, August 24, 1995.
24. These organizations include: The Ministry of Community Development Women Affairs and Children; The Health Education Division of the MOH; Seventh Day Adventist Church Health Services (SDA); The MOH information system unit; The Demographic and Training Unit of the University of Dar es Salaam; The Department of Community Health in the Institute of Public Health at Muhimbili Medical University; The Christian Medical Board of Tanzania (CMBT); *Elimu ya Malezi ya Ujana* (EMAU); The Organization of Tanzania Trade Unions (OTTU); *Chama cha Kitaalamu cha Waalimu cha Tanzania* (CHAKIWATA) (the Tanzania Professional Teachers' Association); The Tanzania Parents Organization (WAZAZI); and the Chama Cha Mapinduzi (CCM).
25. The following internationally based organizations were involved with family planning in Tanzania: The Population Council; Centre for African Family Studies (CAFS); The Programme for International Training in Health (INTRAH); Family Planning Services Expansion and Technical Support Project (SEATS); Family Planning Logistics Management Project (FPLM); Johns Hopkins University Population Communication Services (JHU/PCS); Pathfinder International; Marie Stopes International; and the Association for Voluntary Surgical Contraception (AVSC) now Engender Health.
26. The German Technical Assistance Agency (GTZ) began funding the Family Health Programme in 1980, focusing on acute respiratory infection in children under five and added a family planning/child spacing component in 1987. The Overseas Development Administration of the UK (ODA) now DFID, funded the Mbeya Family Health Project focusing on both public and private provision of health services at the district level. The Norwegian Agency for International Development (NORAD) contributed $0.7 million together with UNFPA funding to establish a family planning "model clinic" for training purposes and a building to house the FPU, now called the Reproductive and Child Health Unit and located at Muhimbili Medical Centre. The Japanese Organization for International Cooperation in Family Planning (JOICFP) sponsored the Integrated Project on Nutrition, Parasite

Control and Family Planning that began in 1983 and that will be discussed in the following chapter.

27. USAID's FPSS provided technical assistance in areas of management, clinical family planning training, logistics, workplace and community-based family planning service provision, and IEC. FPSS also supported national data collection through surveys such as the DHSs, Tanzania Knowledge, Attitude, and Practice Survey, and the Tanzania Situation Analysis, and funded the dissemination of these results to policymakers and health professionals. The project also provided commodities such as clinic equipment and vehicles, as well as almost 60 percent of the contraceptives required by the national program (the other contraceptives were supplied by UNFPA and ODA). It has provided extensive support for the FPU, including hiring personnel, providing equipment, and renting office space. They held trainings for family planning managers, training teams, service providers, and other cadres through a system of regional trainers and health teams. USAID also provided funding through UMATI for developing surgical contraceptive sites and to assist in developing a national training strategy and national curricula for service providers. Through Pathfinder International, USAID has supported workplace and community distribution programs for family planning in conjunction with UMATI, Organization of Tanzania Trade Unions (OTTU), and Tanzanian Occupational Health Services.
28. Countries receiving more aid were (in order): Kenya, Uganda, Ethiopia, Nigeria, Senegal, and Ghana.
29. An USAID informant told me that a meeting of donors in the population and health sectors took place every two months, and a reproductive health coordination and integration group met every month at USAID. When asked if I could have access to any of these meetings or their documents I was told: "These are not open records." I was informed that the government and the Christian Medical Board of Tanzania sent representatives to this coordination group, but that UMATI did not (interview 95DD05, January 29, 1996).
30. Interview 95DD05b, August 5, 1996.
31. Interview 95DD05a, January 29, 1996.
32. Interview 95DD02, December 1, 1995.
33. In a comparison to available information for 16 developing countries over time, there were 8 countries with an increasing dependence on the public sector, 5 countries with an increasing dependence on the private sector, and 3 countries with no change. This study found no correlation between success and privatization (Mauldin and Ross 1989).
34. UMATI notes "If Tanzania is to make a significant change in its current rate of population growth, it will need to move quickly to emphasize the longer term contraceptive methods, especially surgical contraception (UMATI 1992, 4).
35. They note that this is "also an area where government programs are typically reluctant to act (UMATI 1992, 5).
36. Interview 95GR09, August 20, 1996.
37. Interview 95GK30, November 5, 1996.
38. Interview 95GM25a, January 19, 1996.

39. Interview 95GK31, October 22, 1996.
40. The service provider did not even recognize the district coordinator when we arrived so it was clear that they had not had much experience working together before the evaluation visit.
41. Participant observation field notes, 95GK18, November 11, 1996.
42. Participant observation field notes, 95GM10, March 1, 1996.
43. Interview 95GK34, October 18, 1996.
44. Interview 95GK34, October 18, 1996.
45. Interview 95NO08, November 19, 1996.
46. Interview 95NO08, November 19, 1996.
47. Higher levels of infertility in some regions may be partly responsible for the appearance of a lower total fertility rate (Larsen 1997).

Chapter 4 Humanistic Family Planning—Governing Population at the Grassroots

1. The Integrated Project is based on the Japanese experience of providing family planning to rural areas and was first implemented in Taiwan (1975) and in Indonesia, Korea, the Philippines, and Thailand (1976) (Tanzania Food and Nutrition Centre 1995, 2).
2. Other CBD projects have been undertaken by the Ministry of Health (in Tabora, Dodoma, Coast, and Iringa Regions); UMATI (in Dar es Salaam, Coast, Kilimanjaro, Morogoro and Iringa Regions); the Seventh Day Adventist (SDA) Church (in Tabora, Dodoma, Coast, Morogoro and Iringa Regions), and Marie Stopes. Small CBD projects were also implemented at the University of Dar es Salaam, the OTTU, and the field-force unit [*jeshi ya kujenga taifa*] (Mpango wa Taifa wa Uzazi wa Mpango na Afya ya Uzazi 1997, vii).
3. CBD Supervisory Manual, Agency Training Manual, and Training Manual for District Training of Trainers (UMATI 1995a, 4).
4. This is my translation; the text reads: *Mwelekeo huo unalenga katika kuutazama Uzazi wa Mpango kama sehemu ya Afya ya Uzazi.*
5. This number does not correspond with the population statistics found in any documents on the project, so either the IPPF officials were given different numbers—the difference between 8,000 and 15,000 did not matter to the project—or this figure itself is a typographical error.
6. From an untitled 1987 or 1988 document describing the IP in Tanzania located in the "Tanzania" file, IPPF London.
7. In 1988, the project expanded laterally from Roo and Modio to include all six villages of Masama East Ward (population of approximately 23,091 people) and from the TPC to include all four villages of Mabogini Ward. Also in 1988, the project was expanded to a second region, with the introduction of IP in six villages (Bumu, Pinde, Kibaoni, Langali, Lusungi, and Lukuyu) of Mgeta Ward, Morogoro Rural District in Morogoro Region (population of approximately 9,248 people). In 1992, the expansion continued in Masama

to include 47 villages in Hai District with a population coverage of approximately 139,229. By 1995, the IP was in almost all the villages of Hai district and about 10 villages in neighboring Moshi Rural District. The Mgeta site expanded to include another ward down the mountain from Mgeta, Mlali. These five villages (Mlali, Kipera, Manza, Mongwe, and Peko Msegese) have an approximate population of 12,165 people. In 1995, the IP moved to Mwanza Region, where it was initiated in five villages of Magu District.

8. Interview 95NO18, May 5, 1996.
9. Interview 95NO10, March 5, 1996.
10. Percentages of infected children were 14 percent in project areas and 8.7 percent in nonproject areas with a p-value of 0.01214 noted as "highly significant" (Tanzania Food and Nutrition Centre 1995, 41).
11. Interview 95NO08, November 19, 1996.
12. Interview 95NO13, October 17, 1996.
13. "Prior to 1993, the emphasis of the strategy for this project was on increasing family planning delivery points. On the contrary, from 1993 the emphasis was changed to increasing the Couple Year of Protection (CYP) in selected rural and urban marginal populations through the provision of high quality, comprehensive, accessible, and client responsive family planning services. . . ." (Mkini 1995, 4).
14. By the time of my earliest work in the village, the car had broken down and a replacement had not been sent. Participant observation field notes 95GM14, May 7, 1996.
15. Participant observation field notes 95NO12, December 17, 1995.
16. Interview 95GD02, September 12, 1995.
17. Interview 95NO17, March 15, 1996.
18. Interview 95NO13, October 17, 1996.
19. Personal communication, 95GM14, May 7, 1996.
20. Interview 95NO18, May 5, 1996.
21. One particular example is from the brick-making project in one village. I was shown the pile of bricks to be cooked to demonstrate the non-family planning activities of the CBDs. These bricks, I was told, were to be used to build an UMATI office and a nursery school in the village. However, as months passed and the bricks were never moved, I asked about the planned building and was told that it was just about to begin "next week." Another informant suggested that there had been some confusion by one of the local project leaders over whether these bricks were an UMATI project or his own personal income-generating project. A similar problem was related to me "off the record" regarding a different project component, and another one involved a visit by the local police to one of the project leader's houses.
22. From participant observation fieldnotes, 95NO12 7/17/95.
23. "*Usimpe samaki – umfundishe kuvua samaki.*" Participant observation fieldnotes 95GM14, July 3, 1996.
24. Participant observation field notes 95GM14, July 3, 1996.
25. Participant observation field notes 95GM14, July 3, 1996.
26. Interview 95NO15, October 14, 1996.
27. CBD Interview 95NO16, May 3, 1996.

28. This same issue of the nursery school funding was brought up at the meeting of the local steering committee. The UMATI representative asked the CBDs if they knew why the villagers would not pay the fees, suggesting that perhaps the school was not providing a good service. One person spoke up and said that there had been a flier posted around the village saying that the nursery school was an UMATI school, so everyone thought that it was free. From field notes, 95GM14, March 5, 1996.
29. This is particularly relevant in areas where there are different projects operating simultaneously. I was told by an informant that UMATI had chosen to train CBDs in one village who had already been trained by another community-based health project. Because the UMATI CBDs were given bicycles as incentives, the workers in the other project who were not also UMATI affiliates complained that they were not being appropriately compensated. Interview 95NO13, October 17, 1996.
30. Interview 95DD05a, January 29, 1996.
31. Interview 95NO14, March 4, 1996.
32. At the Local Steering Committee meeting I attended, participants received a per diem of 8,000 Tsh ($13.50). To put this in perspective, the average family net farm income in this village was approximately 138,000 Tsh ($230) per year (Ponte 2002).
33. Interview 95NO08, November 19, 1996.
34. Furthermore, the UMATI manager who was to become the project supervisor had attended a closing ceremony of a training seminar in the village the previous week, yet she did not even introduce herself to the local CBDs in attendance (participant observation 95GM14, July 3, 1996).
35. These meetings are supposed to be held four times per year to run the local project.
36. All data in this section come from participant observation 95GM14, July 3, 1996.
37. For a critique of the notion of "expertise" from a gender perspective see Parpart (1995).
38. This reminds us that notions of women's empowerment can mask power relations between different categories of women (see Yuval-Davies 1994 cited in Rowlands 1998), and that we must integrate women as well as gender into our analysis (see Jackson 1998).
39. The use of incentives has been called into question for both its incompatibility with a user perspective that believes in client's rights, and for its management consequences for health sector workers; see for example Staudt (1991).
40. From participant observation, 95GM14, May 7, 1996.
41. From participant observation, 95NO12, July 17, 1995.
42. From participant observation , 95NO12, July 12, 1995.
43. He linked passive acceptors with the expansion of family planning to include a larger reproductive health agenda. This may suggest a self-conscious attempt to integrate a women's empowerment agenda with demographic and development agendas.
44. From participant observation, 95NO12, July 12, 1995.

Intermezzo 2 Development in Theater and Practice: The Regional Workshop on the Integrated Project

1. Invited delegates came from Cameroon, Ethiopia, the Gambia, Ghana, Guinea (Conakry), Kenya, Madagascar, Nigeria, Senegal, Sierra Leone, Tanzania, Togo, Uganda, and Zambia.
2. From the "Participants List for the Regional Workshop on the Integrated Project (PANFRICO V) in Dar es Salaam Tanzania, 5–11 December 1995."
3. I was particularly curious when I saw a large group of men in tuxedos sitting to the side of the podium. I quickly found out that they were members of a brass band hired to play during workshop breaks while participants ate hors d'oeuvres.
4. "Medicines" probably referred to contraceptives in light of the shortage in supplies of deworming medicines.
5. I was informed by the group coordinator that because we were running extremely late, he had sent down money to supply the musicians with local beer to maintain their enthusiasm while waiting for the group.
6. Ethically, it seems inconceivable that a rural woman defined as a "family planning acceptor" would be displayed in her home for two buses full of development tourists to ask her questions about intimate aspects of her life.

Chapter 5 Identities, Expectations, and Control: Negotiating Traditional Practices and Modern Methods

1. See for example Bordo (1990); Ginsburg and Rapp (1995); Jacobus, Keller et al. (1990); Lykke and Braidotti (1996); Yanoshik and Norsigian (1989).
2. It is important to note that I am discussing both modern and traditional methods in the framework of the international population discourse as embodied by the National Family Planning Programme that is itself a modern construct emphasizing modern methods. The informants in this research are all engaging in knowledge production from a modern bias. I did not interview traditional healers (*Waganga*), nor did I seek out women who had long experiences using traditional methods.
3. As listed in the report, these are: status and prestige attained by having children; having many children confirms one's virtue; self-image enhanced by producing children; a man's lineage is continued through his children; proof that one has been favored by spiritual forces and deceased ancestors; short-term economic gain provided by children through farm labor; long-term economic gain provided by children by caring for parents when they are old; lack of forward planning and belief in fatalism; polygamy; taboo against husband and wife discussing sexual matters; fostering children; early marriage for

women; infant mortality and the fear of children dying or becoming disabled (USAID 1990, 61,62).

4. Interview 95GD02, September 12, 1995.
5. Interview 95GR30, September 21, 1996. While Tanzanian policymakers did not try to explain why this had happened, women from Lusewa, told me that when education became mandatory, they could no longer hold the same initiation ceremonies to pass on teachings as they had in the past. Other works such as Van Eeuwijk and Mlangwa (1997) and Tumbo-Masabo (1994) describe the gap between the initiation ceremonies and modern education about sexuality in Tanzania.
6. "[Hu]man-made" traditional contraceptive devices described by my respondents included herbs to ingest and tying a string around the waist. Ntukula includes the use of a piece of cloth inserted into the vagina before intercourse and covering a pot symbolic of a woman's fertility (1994, 112).
7. Interview 95NO10, March 5, 1996.
8. Interview 95GM24a, July 12, 1996.
9. This was an explanation given by a rural service provider for the increasing number of women "choosing" to be sterilized. Interview 00GK02, October 6, 2000.
10. Adeokun (1991) notes that "most of the key terms used in family planning carry both ordinary and specialized meanings" which can be confusing to service providers and the general public. He gives an anecdote from a physician who told of a woman who had introduced a bedspring coil into her vagina in the mistaken belief that she was adopting the IUD, also known as the "coil." Other terms he mentions with multiple meanings are "pills" and "injection." These problems are exponentially increased when terminology is taken from one language to another.
11. Also, important policy documents such as the "National Policy Guidelines and Standards for Family Planning Service Delivery and Training" that I observed in regional MCH offices and the "Client-Oriented Provider-Efficient Services: A Process and Tools for Quality Improvement in Family Planning and Other Reproductive Health Services" (1995) which was available at an NGO clinic were in English as well.
12. Different standards explain why women in rural Tanzania can receive oral contraceptive pills from their neighbours after responding to a checklist of questions, while women in the West are likely to have them prescribed during a visit to a medical doctor.
13. Normally, I declined offers to observe invasive medical procedures as I felt that even with consent it was not appropriate for my research. My presence in this moment was accidental: the same space was used for a number of activities, and I had been talking with another service provider on a bench on the other side of the room. When I realized that they had instructed the young woman to prepare herself for a pelvic exam, my dilemma was over whether to get up, explain my departure, and leave the room, which would require opening the only door that led to a crowded waiting area and would expose the room to others, or to stay put and try to be as unobtrusive as possible. I chose the latter.
14. Interview 00GK03, November 29, 2000.

15. Johnson-Hanks 2002 makes a similar argument for Cameroon.
16. Interview 20905, September 19, 1996.
17. Interview 17120, June 15, 1996.
18. Interview 20818, October 1, 1996.

Chapter 6 Contraceptive Technologies for Planning Local Families

1. In Uganda, for comparison, in line with the concept introduced at the Cairo conference, the Maternal and Child Health/Family Planning Department was renamed in 1999 to become the Reproductive Health Division (Uganda Ministry of Health 2000), which produced the "Sexual and Reproductive Health Minimum Package for Uganda" (Uganda Ministry of Health 1999).
2. Luke and Watkins' (2002) study of national elites in Ghana, Bangladesh, Malawi, Senegal, and Jordan found that respondents in all countries supported family planning and maternal health programs, but tended to pick and choose among the other components promoted at Cairo. Bangser (1999) notes that Tanzanian managers and planners are concerned that they are unjustly evaluated against an externally created and imposed "ICPD checklist."
3. According to TDHS and TRCHS data, 90.5 percent of all Tanzanian women were using no method in 1992; 83.9 percent in 1996; and 77.7 percent in 1999.
4. The famous "KAP gap" [knowledge, attitude, and practice] as it is termed in demographic literature.
5. Given that the national mean for ideal number of children was six according to the DHS at the time of the interviews, it seemed reasonable that many women who were neither pregnant nor postpartum would not be using contraception because they would want to become pregnant.
6. There were small but expected differences by region, since these regions were purposively selected for diversity, with 83 percent of women having used contraception in Kilimanjaro; 74 percent in Morogoro and 73 percent in Ruvuma regions.
7. This table is somewhat awkward reflecting the difficulties of translating the narrative terms in which women told their contraceptive histories into the frozen slice-in-time terms in which we analyze them. Women were asked if they had ever used any method of family planning, then they were asked questions about that method, and finally they were asked if they were still using the method and if not, why they stopped and if they ever again used another method.
8. The percentage of women whose partners were using condoms as their first contraceptive was even greater for urban areas. For example, in Morogoro, 43 percent of women used condoms compared to 34 percent using pills.
9. I should clarify that this was often before marriage to a man, whom they later married. The onset of family planning use was still more often after having proven fertility.
10. Interview 17180, December 1, 1996.

11. See the work of Setel 1995 for an anthropological investigation of the perceptions of AIDS in Kilimanjaro.
12. Reflections on interviews 31109 and 31111, November 4, 1996.
13. All names used are pseudonyms.
14. From Oxford's Standard Swahili-English Dictionary.
15. I thank Frances Vavrus for her insight into this interpretation.
16. This of course also reflects my perception that women who had previously had an unwanted pregnancy would be more likely to use contraception afterward. However, the other scenario is that women who were "good planners" with wanted children are those most likely to be using contraception successfully.
17. Despite the different definitions of "marriage" according to different cultural groups and to the legal union under the state and/or church, I am using "marriage" to include anyone who self-identified as married, which includes those women who were living together with a man in a "marriage-like" relationship.
18. From my data, the median age of the mother at the first conception was 18, with expected regional variation of 19 in Kilimanjaro, 18 in Morogoro, and 17 in Ruvuma.
19. In Tanzanian "health education," women are taught that they should not begin childbearing until age 20. In spite of studies showing that maternal age ceases to exert an independent effect on birth outcomes (Geronimus 1987; 1994; Makinson 1985) or that the effect may be in the opposite direction, that is, young mothers in some contexts have better birth outcomes (Geronimus 1994), "adolescent pregnancy" (before age 20) has become an international development category of "high risk" birth to be avoided.
20. Conversely, infertility is a dramatic aberration in one's personhood. Allen (2004) describes how fears of infertility have a profound effect on the health-seeking behavior of Tanzanian women and their families.
21. Allen (2004) also documents instances of successful and unsuccessful induced abortion during her time of residence in a rural Shinyanga community.
22. This chronicled every pregnancy that each woman had experienced and the result of that pregnancy.
23. As it was not central to my interests, I did not ask about it directly, although I tried to ask follow-up questions whenever women themselves initiated the topic.
24. In the larger socioeconomic context of the household and community, this may also relate to a general perception that life is becoming more difficult. As I will discuss later in this chapter, survey data from Machame, a wealthy rural community suggest that this is the case.
25. Of course, it also means that these women experienced some form of contraceptive failure, since we were discussing method use in the context of pregnancies they had conceived.
26. As described in chapter six, there was a common practice in this area of abstaining from sexual practices that would risk the mixing of semen and

breast milk inside a woman's body as this was thought to bring harm to the breastfeeding child.

27. For comparison, Hayes (1987) argues that for the case of African-American teenage mothers "marriage only worsens a pregnant girl's situation: it increases her chances of closely spaced pregnancies, decreases her chances of ever returning to school, and cuts her off from childcare help from family and thus a chance to work, while pairing her with a man whose financial prospects are fragile at best" (cited in Ward 1995, 155).
28. This has not always been the case. One respondent explained to me that in 1993 after hearing the health education talks at the clinic about family planning, she went home to talk to her husband. "If you didn't bring a letter [from your husband], you couldn't get family planning."
29. These findings are quite different from the in-depth interviews of the Nyanza Province study in which the question was asked, "who makes the decision about family planning?" and the predominant response was "the men do" (Watkins, Rutenberg, and Wilkinson 1997, 233). One explanation of difference here may be that the Nyanza respondents were speaking of family planning decision making in general, while my respondents were speaking from their own experience during the first time they used contraception. Thus, the women in Nyanza related information about the community norm, while my respondents were explaining their own experiences. Another explanation may come from the fact that all of my respondents to this question had used family planning, so it may be that they engaged in decision-making patterns more likely to lead to contraceptive use, and that women who would have agreed that the men make these decisions had never used family planning, and thus are not represented in my analysis here.
30. I conducted in-depth interviews with married couples who had previously responded to my household survey in Machame Division, Kilimanjaro Region.
31. The MCH/FP clinics in Tanzania are highly "feminized" spaces (Booth 1995) where men are only found as a result of dire circumstances such as a seriously ill child.
32. Men's abdication of economic responsibility for their children is nothing new. Turshen describes how the custom of married women assuming economic responsibility for themselves and their children can be traced to the absence of men resulting from slavery, and persisting throughout colonialism's transition to the capitalist mode of production (1987, 191). While colonialists found it advantageous to pay only a single man's wage, African men too found it advantageous to believe their women to be self-supporting. Turshen suggests that African men continued to expect their wives to assume the economic burden of children in an attempt to preserve their power over the women (Ibid.).
33. Interview 31018, November 1, 1996.
34. The increasing levels of differentiation, and decreasing access to public services for the poor may affect the perceived "costs" of children as has been argued for the case of Kenya (see Buckley 1998; Dow, Archer, Khasiani, and Kekovole 1994; Watkins 1998).

35. In practice, most of these fears seemed unfounded and husbands were quite willing to talk to me at length on these issues during in-depth interviews. This may be attributable to the fact that I had become familiar to many of the community members and that I was visibly pregnant myself when I conducted this research, a fact to which most of my respondents referred.
36. Using a questionnaire in Swahili, local assistants trained in interviewing and survey techniques and I conducted a household survey in Machame. A total of 254 households were interviewed, but available data are sometimes slightly fewer. The project is entitled "Methods, Meanings and Measurements in Contraceptive Decision-Making" hereafter referred to as the 3M project.

Chapter 7 Conclusion

1. A health education poster in urban clinics tries to promote condoms as a family planning method for married couples with children, noting both that condoms have no side effects for parents or their children and that they also prevent sexually transmitted diseases including HIV/AIDS. However, while some research suggests that condoms are becoming more widely used in nonmarital sexual encounters, they continue to be unacceptable within marriage (Kapiga and Lugalla 2002).
2. I began to notice the limited method provision as early as 2000 in the clinics in the district where I worked.
3. When I asked at a few clinics where these methods were popular in the past I was either told that they did not have the supplies anymore, or that they no longer had a trained doctor, or in one case, that they do them but not regularly.
4. The concept of unmet need serves to link the reproductive health agenda and the population control ideology. Deconstructing this problematic concept goes far beyond the scope of this chapter, but in brief, unmet need has been used to show that governments can achieve demographic goals by simply focusing on satisfying the existing demand for fertility regulation, and thus explicit targets are no longer necessary. This conclusion reassured governments that "it was possible to achieve demographic goals without pursuing numbers-driven population policies" (Casterline and Sinding 2000). Unmet need is used to defend the central role of family planning even within a larger agenda of reproductive health.
5. Malthus' model of population as an endogenous variable where birth and death rates vary in response to changes in the standard of living was foundational in placing food availability at the centre of the population scare.
6. For a clear illustration of demographic concepts such as transition theory see Crook and Timæus 1997.
7. The world population growth rate peaked in the 1960s and then began declining. Explanations for declining growth rates vary by geographical context, but usually include some combination of social and economic advances, expanding education and employment for women, and access to family planning programs.

8. This suggests the uncritical perpetuation of the persistent myth of Africa as a development basket case (see for example the case made by Zeleza 1997).
9. In a footnote, Cohen refers to another work that mentions HIV infection as a risk for young women who use sexual relations for economic support. Interestingly, AIDS is found in the discussion of licentious African sexual behavior, but not in its impact on fertility or demographic shifts.
10. However, Riley and McCarthy (2003) argue that is has had almost no impact, and there were many speculations arising around the time of Cairo; for example see Cleland 1996; Finkle and McIntosh 1996; Potts 1995; van de Kaa 1996 for the negative response and Presser and Sen 2000 for the positive one.
11. Some of whom are also demographers.
12. For an interesting analysis of how Western experts are exporting our obsession with "risk" in childbirth see Ginsburg and Rapp 1995.

Bibliography

Abernethy, V. (1993) *Population Politics: The Choices that Shape our Future.* New York: Insight Books.

Adeokun, L.A. (1991). "Contraception and quality of care in Sub-Saharan Africa: application and extension of a framework." In IUSSP Committee on Comparative Analysis of Fertility and University of Zimbabwe Seminar on The Course of Fertility Transition in Sub-Saharan Africa. Harare, Zimbabwe.

Afshar, H and Dennis, C. (1992). *Women and Adjustment Policies in the Third World.* London, Macmillian.

Akerele, C.O. (1985). "Health Services and Development: Population Issues." In *Fallout from the Population Explosion.* Ed. Villee C.A Jr. New York: Paragon House Publishers. pp. 59–70.

Allen, D.R. (2004) *Managing Motherhood, Managing Risk: Fertility and Danger in West Central Tanzania.* Ann Arbor: University of Michigan Press.

(AMMP) Ministry of Health and AMMP Team (1997). *Policy Implications of Adult Morbidity and Mortality.* End of Phase 1 Report. Technical Report No. 1. Dar es Salaam, United Republic of Tanzania, Ministry of Health/ AMMP Team.

Anagnost, A. (1995). "A Surfeit of Bodies: Population and the Rationality of the State in Post-Mao China." In *Conceiving the New World Order: The Global Politics of Reproduction.* Eds. Faye, Ginsburg, and Rapp. Berkeley: University of California. pp. 22–41.

———. 2004. "The Corporeal Politics of Quality (Suzhi)." *Public Culture* 16(2):189–208.

Apffel-Marglin, F. (1996). "Rationality, the Body, and the World: From Production to Regeneration." In *Decolonizing Knowledge: From Development to Dialogue.* Ed. Apffel-Marglin, F. and S.A. Marglin. Oxford: Clarendon Press. pp. 142–181.

Appadurai, A. (1991). "Global Ethnoscapes: Notes and Queries for a Transnational Anthropology." In *Recapturing Anthropology: Working in the Present.* Ed. R.G. Fox. Santa Fe, New Mexico: School of American Research Advanced Seminar Series. pp. 191–210.

Ashford, L.S. (2001). "New Population Policies: Advancing Women's Health and Rights." *Population Bulletin* 56(1) March : accessed online at http://www.prb.org/Publications/PopulationBulletins.aspx on September 10, 2007.

Askew, Ian and Marge Berer. (2003). "The Contribution of Sexual and Reproductive Health Services to the Fight against HIV/AIDS: A Review." *Reproductive Health Matters* 11 (22):51–73.

Azefor, M. (1988). *Policies and Family Planning Programs in Africa: Evaluation and Prospects in African Population*. Leige: IUSSP.

Bandarage, A. (1997). *Women, Population and Global Crisis*. London and New Jersey: Zed Books.

Bangser, M. (1999). "Tanzania Promoting Reproductive Health; Investing in Health for Development." In *Promoting Reproductive Health: Investing in Health for Development*. Ed. Forman, S., R. Ghosh. Boulder, CO and London: Lynne Rienner. pp. 183–220.

Barrett, D.A. (1995). "Reproducing Persons as a Global Concern: The Making of An Institution." PhD Dissertation, Department of Sociology, Stanford University.

Barrett, D. and D.J. Frank. (1999). "Population Control for National Development: From World Discourse to National Policies." In *Constructing World Culture: International Nongovernmental Organizations Since 1875*. Ed. Boli, J. and G.M. Thomas. Stanford, CA: Stanford University Press. pp. 198–221.

Barrett, D. and O.A. Tsui. (1999). "Policy as Symbolic Statement: International Response to National Population Policies." *Social Forces* 78(1):213–234.

Baudrillard, J. (1981). *For a Critique of the Political Economy of the Sign*. Translated by Levin, C. St Louis, Mo: Telos Press.

Baylies, C. and J. Bujra. (2000). "Editorial: Special Issue on AIDS." *Review of African Political Economy* (86):483–486.

Begus, S. (1998). "Contentious Contraception: Feminist Debates about the Use of Long-Acting Hormonal Contraceptives by Adolescent Urban Women." In *Daring to Be Good: Essays in Feminist Ethico-Politics*. Eds. Bar On, B.A. and Ferguson, A. New York and London: Routledge. pp. 208–223.

Beneria, L. and S. Feldman. (1992). *Unequal Burden: Economic Crises, Persistent Poverty and Women's Work*. Boulder, CO: Westview Press.

Birdsall, N., A.C. Kelley, and S.W. Sinding. (2001). *Population Matters: Demographic Change, Economic Growth, and Poverty in the Developing World*. New York: Oxford University Press.

Black, J.K. (1991). *Development in Theory and Practice: Bridging the Gap*. Boulder, CO: Westview Press.

Bledsoe, C. (1994). "Constructing Natural Fertility, the use of western contraceptive technologies in rural Gambia," *Population and Development Review* (20): 81–113.

Bledsoe, C.H. (2002). *Contingent Lives: Fertility, Time and Aging in West Africa*. Chicago and London: University of Chicago Press.

Bledsoe, C.H., F. Banja, and A. Hill. (1998). "Reproductive Mishaps and Western Contraception: An African Challenge to Fertility Theory." *Population and Development Review*. 24(1):15–57.

Booth, Karen M. (2004). *Local Women, Global Science: Fighting AIDS in Kenya*. Bloomington and Indianapolis: Indiana Univ. Press.

Bordo, S. (1990). "Reading the Slender Body." In *Body/Politics: Women and the Discourses of Science*. Ed. Jacobus, M., E.F. Keller, and S. Shuttleworth. New York and London: Routledge. pp. 83–112.

Boserup, E. (1970). *Women's Role in Economic Development*. New York: St. Martin's Press.

Bourdieu, P. (1999). *The Weight of the World: Social Suffering in Contemporary Society*. Stanford, California: Stanford University Press.

Boyce, J.K. (2002). "Unpacking Aid." *Development and Change*, 33 (2) April, pp. 239–246.

———. (1991). *Language and Symbolic Power*. Cambridge, Mass.: Harvard University Press.

Brigg, M. (2002). "Foucault and the Colonisation Metaphor." *Third World Quarterly* 23(3):421–436.

Brown, L.R., G. Gardner, and B. Halweil. (1998). *Beyond Malthus: Sixteen Dimensions of the Population Problem*, September, Worldwatch paper #143.

Brush, P. (1998). "Metaphors of Inscription: Discipline, Plasticity and the Rhetoric of Choices." *Feminist Review*. Spring(58):22–43.

Buckley, S. (1998). "Taking a New Line on Families." *Washington Post National Weekly Edition* May 4, 1998, pp. 18.

Bulatao, R. 1993. *Effective Family Planning Programs*. Washington, D.C.: The World Bank.

Bureau of Statistics, Planning Commission, and the EVALUATION Project. (1997). *Tanzania Service Availability Survey 1996*. Dar es Salaam, Tanzania: Bureau of Statistics, Planning Commission.

Cagatay, N., D. Elson, and C. Grown. (1995). "Introduction: Gender, Adjustment and Macroeconomics." *World Development Special Issue* 23(11):1827–1836.

Caldwell, J.C. (1968). "Population Policy: A Survey of Commonwealth Africa." In *The Population of Tropical Africa*. Ed. Caldwell, J.C. and C. Okonjo. London: Longman. pp. 368–375.

Calhoun, Craig. (2003). "Why Historical Sociology." In *Handbook of Historical Sociology*. Eds. Delanty, Gerard and Engin Isin. London: Sage. pp. 383–395.

Carpenter, L. M., J. S. Nakiyingi, A. Ruberantwari, S. Malamba, A. Kamali, and J.A.G. Whitworth. (1997). "Estimates of the Impact of HIV Infection on Fertility in a Rural Ugandan Population Cohort." *Health Transition Review* 7(suppl 2):113–126.

Casterline, J.B. and S.W. Sinding. (2000). "Unmet Need for Family Planning in Developing Countries and Implications for Population Policy." *Population and Development Review* 26(4):691–723.

Chambers, R. (1983). *Rural Development: Putting the Last First*. Harlow: Longman.

Chatterjee, N. and N.E. Riley. (2001). "Planning an Indian Modernity: The Gendered Politics of Fertility Control." *Signs: Journal of Women in Culture and Society* 26(3):811–845.

Chavkin, W. and E. Chesler, eds. (2005). *Where Human Rights Begin: Health, Sexuality, and Women in the New Millennium*. New Brunswick, NJ. and London: Rutgers University Press.

Chen, S. and D.K. Guilkey. (2003). "Determinants of Contraceptive Method Choice in Rural Tanzania Between 1991 and 1999." *MEASURE Evaluation Working Paper*. WP-03–75 Chapel Hill, NC: MEASURE Evaluation.

Chesler, E. (2005). "Introduction." In *Where Human Rights Begin: Essays on Health, Sexuality and Women, Ten Years after Vienna, Cairo and Beijing*. Ed. W. Chavkin and E. Chesler. New Brunwick, NJ and London: Rutgers University Press. pp. 1–34.

Clarke, A.E. and V.L. Olesen, eds. (1999). *Revisioning Women, Health and Healing: Feminist, Cultural, and Technoscience Perspectives*. New York and London: Routledge.

Cleland, J. and C. Scott, eds. (1987). *The World Fertility Survey: An Assessment of Its Contribution*. Oxford: Oxford University Press.

Cleland, J. (1996). "ICPD and the Feminization of Population and Development Issues." *Heath Transition Review* 6:107–110.

Cohen, B. (1998). "The Emerging Fertility Transition in Sub-Saharan Africa." *World Development* 26(8):1431–1461.

———. (2000). "Family Planning Programs, Socioeconomic Characteristics, and Contraceptive Use in Malawi." *World Development* 28(5):843–860.

Cooper, F. and Packard, R. (1997). "Introduction." In *International Development and the Social Sciences: Essays on the History and Politics of Knowledge*. Ed. Cooper, F. and R. Packard. Berkeley: University of California Press. pp. 1–44.

Crook, N. and I. Timæus. (1997). *Principles of Population and Development with Illustrations from Asia and Africa*. Oxford: Oxford University Press.

Cruikshank, B. (1999). *The Will to Empower: Democratic Citizens and Other Subjects*, Ithaca and London: Cornell University Press.

Cuffaro, N. (1997). "Population Growth and Agriculture in Poor Countries: A Review of Theoretical Issues and Empirical Evidence." *World Development* 25(7):1151–1163.

Curtis, C. (1989). "Declaring War on Worms in Tanzania." *People*. London: International Planned Parenthood Federation.

Delany, S.R. (1994). "The Rhetoric of Sex, the Discourse of Desire." In *Heterotopia: Postmodern Utopia and the Body Politic*. Ed. Siebers, T. Ann Arbor: University of Michigan Press. pp. 229–272.

Desrosières, A. (1998). *The Politics of Large Numbers: A History of Statistical Reasoning*. Translated by Naish, C. Cambridge, Mass.: Harvard University Press.

De Waal, A. (2003). "How Will HIV/AIDS Transform African Governance?" *African Affairs* (102):1–23.

di Leonardo, M. (1998). *Exotics at Home*. Chicago: University of Chicago Press.

Disney, Richard. (2002). "Africa in Crisis: Hazards Rise for Prime-Age Adults" on ID21 Communicating Development Research, May 31. http://www.id21.org/zinter/id21zinter.exe?a=2&i=Insights42art3&u=46e80b4a accessed on September 10, 2007.

Dixon-Mueller, R. and A. Germain. (2000). "Reproductive Health and the Demographic Imagination." In *Women's Empowerment and Demographic Processes: Moving Beyond Cairo*. Eds. Presser, H.B. and G. Sen. Oxford: Oxford University Press. pp. 69–94.

Dow, T.E. Jr., L. Archer, S. Khasiani, and J. Kekovole. (1994). "Wealth Flow and Fertility Decline in Rural Kenya." *Population and Development Review* 20(2):343–363.

Duden, B. (1993). "Population." In *The Development Dictionary: A Guide to Knowledge as Power.* Ed. Sachs, W. London: Zed Press, pp. 72–76.

du Lou, A., P. Msellati, et al. (1999). "Impaired Fertility in HIV-1 Infected Pregnant Women: A Clinic-Based Survey in Abidjan, Cote d'Ivoire." *AIDS* 13: 517–521.

Durkheim, E. (1961) [1915]. *The Elementary Forms of the Religious Life.* New York: Collier.

Dye, T.R. (1972). *Understanding Public Policy.* Englewood Cliffs, NJ: Prentice-Hall.

ECA Population Division. (1982). "Fifth Population Inquiry Among Governments: ECA Member States Perceptions and Policies on Demographic Trends in Relation to Development as of 1982." ECA Population Division.

Eckstein, H. (1975). "Case Study and Theory in Political Science." In *Handbook of Political Science* Vol. 7. Eds. Greenstein, F and N.W. Polsby. New York: Addison-Wesley.

Ekanem, I.I. (1988). "African Population Policies: Formulation and Implementation in the 1970s and 1980s." In *African Population Conference Dakar 1988, (3)* Dakar, Senegal: International Union for the Scientific Study of Population. pp. 1–17.

Elson, D. (1995). "Gender Awareness in Modeling Structural Adjustment." *World Development* 23(11):1851–1868.

———. (1991). "Male Bias in Macro-Economics: The Case of Structural Adjustment. Male" In *Bias in the Development Process.* Ed. Elson, D. Manchester: Manchester University Press. pp. 164–190.

Erlich, P.R. (1968). *The Population Bomb.* New York: Ballentine.

Erlich, P.R. and A.H. Erlich. (1990). *The Population Explosion.* New York: Simon and Schuster.

Family Planning Unit, Tanzanian Ministry of Health. (1992). "National Family Planning Programme: Background, Status of Activities, Strengths and Constraints." Presented to the FP Participating Agencies Meeting held at Morogoro Hotel, February 12–14, 1992. Morogoro, Tanzania.

Farmer, P. (1999). *Infections and Inequalities: The Modern Plagues.* Berkeley: University of California Press.

Feeney, G. (2001). 'The Impact of HIV/AIDS on Adult Mortality in Zimbabwe.' *Population and Development Review* 27(4):771–780.

Ferguson, J. (1999). *Expectations of Modernity: Myths and Meanings of Urban Life on the Zambian Copperbelt.* Berkeley: University of California Press.

———. (1997). "Anthropology and Its Evil Twin: 'Development' in the Constitution of a Discipline." In *International Development and the Social Sciences: Essays on the History and Politics of Knowledge.* Ed. Cooper, F and R. Packard. Berkeley: University of California Press. pp. 150–175.

———. (1994). *The Anti-Politics Machine: "Development," Depoliticization, and Bureaucratic Power in Lesotho.* Minneapolis and London: University of Minnesota Press.

Finkle, J.L. and A. McIntosh. (1996). "Cairo Revisited: Some Thoughts on the Implications of the ICPD." *Health Transition Review* 6:110–113.

Finkle, J.L. and B.B. Crane, (1975). "The Politics of Bucharest: Population, Development and the New International Economic Order." *Population and Development Review* 1(1):87–114.

Finkle, J.L. (1985). "Ideology and Politics at Mexico City: The United States at the 1984 International Conference on Population." *Population and Development Review* 11(1):1–28.

Firestone, S. (1970). *The Dialectic of Sex: The Case for Feminist Revolution.* New York: William and Morrow, Co.

Fisher, Kate and Simon Szreter. (2003). "'They Prefer Withdrawal': The Choice of Birth Control in Britain, 1918–1950." *Journal of Interdisciplinary History* 34(2), Autumn:263–291.

Foucault, M. (1980). *The History of Sexuality Volume I: An Introduction.* New York: Vintage Books.

———. (1979). *Discipline and Punish: The Birth of the Prison.* New York: Vintage Books.

Freedman, L.P. (1999). "Censorship and Manipulation of Family Planning Information: An Issue of Human Rights and Women's Health." In *Health and Human Rights.* Ed. Mann, S. Gruskin, S. Grodin, M.A.and G.J. Annas, G.J. New York and London: Routledge. pp. 145–178.

Fukuda, T. (2005). *Community Operated Reproductive Health.* JOICFP. Tokyo, www.joicfp.or.jp accessed on June 9, 2005.

Furedi, F. (1997). *Population and Development: A Critical Introduction.* New York: St. Martin's Press.

George, A. (1979). "Case Studies and Theory Development: The Method of Structured Focused Comparison." In *Diplomatic History: New Approaches.* Ed. Lauren, P.G. New York: Free Press. pp. 43–68.

Geronimus, A. (1994). "The Weathering Hypothesis and the Health of African-American Women and Infants: Implications for Reproductive Strategies and Policy Analysis." In *Power and Decision: The Social Control of Reproduction.* Ed. Sen, G and R.C. Snow. Boston: Harvard Center for Population and Development Studies. pp. 77–100.

Geronimus, A. (1987). "On Teenage Childbearing and Neonatal Mortality in the United States." *Population and Development Review* 13:245–279.

Gibbon, P. (1991). Population and Poverty in the Changing Ideology of the World Bank. *Population and the Development Crisis in the South.* M. Hammarskjold. Lund, Sweden, Program on Population and Development in Poor Countries, University of Lund.

Ginsburg, F.D. and R. Rapp. (1995). "Introduction: Conceiving the New World Order." In *Conceiving the New World Order: The Global Politics of Reproduction.* Ed. Ginsburg and Rapp. Berkeley: University of California Press. pp. 1–17.

Gladwin, C.H., ed. (1991). *Structural Adjustment and African Women Farmers.* Gainesville, FL: University of Florida Press.

Goppel, W.H. (1987). "Workshop on Population and Development for Party Members." UNFPA.

Green, M. (2000). "Public Reform and the Privatisation of Poverty: Some Institutional Determinants of Health Seeking Behavior in Southern Tanzania." *Culture, Medicine and Psychiatry* 24:403–430.

Greenhalgh, S. (1995) "Anthropology Theorizes Reproduction: Integrating Practice, Political Economic, and Feminist Perspectives." In *Situating Fertility: Anthropology and Demographic Inquiry.* Ed. S. Greenhalgh. Cambridge: Cambridge University Press. pp. 3–28.

Gregson, S., B. Zaba, et al. (1999). "Low Fertility in Women with HIV and the Impact of the Epidemic on Orphanhood and Early Childhood Mortality in Sub-Saharan Africa." *AIDS* 13(suppl A):249–257.

Grewal, I. and C. Kaplan. (1994). *Scattered Hegemonies: Postmodernity and Transnational Feminist Practices.* Minneapolis, MN: University of Minnesota Press.

Grimes, D. and A. Arowojolu. (2003). "Clinical Challenges." *Network, Family Health International* 22(3):17–19.

Grindle, M.S., and J.W. Thomas. (1991). *Public Choices and Policy Change, The Political Economy of Reform in Developing Countries.* Baltimore and London: The Johns Hopkins University Press.

Grosz, E. (1994). *Volatile Bodies: Towards a Corporeal Feminism.* Australia: Allen and Unwin.

Habermas, J. (2005). "Equal Treatment of Cultures and the Limits of Postmodern Liberalism." *The Journal of Political Philosophy* 13(1):1–28.

Hansen, Lene. (2006). *Security as Practice: Discourse Analysis and the Bosnian War.* New York and London: Routledge.

Haraway, D.J. (1991). *Simians, Cyborgs, and Women: The Reinvention of Nature.* New York and London: Routledge.

Harcourt, W. (1999). "Reproductive Health and Rights and the Quest for Social Justice." (Editorial) *Development* 42(1):7–10.

Harrison, G. (2001). "Reform: Reflections on the Cases of Uganda and Tanzania." *Development and Change* (32):657–679.

Hartmann, B. (1995). *Reproductive Rights and Wrongs: The Global Politics of Population Control.* Boston: South End Press.

Hartouni, V. (1997). *Cultural Conceptions: On Reproductive Technologies and the Remaking of Life.* Minneapolis: University of Minnesota Press.

Harvey, D. (2001). *Spaces of Capital : Towards a Critical Geography.* New York: Routledge,

Hayes, C.D. (1987). *Risking the Future: Adolescent Sexuality, Pregnancy, and Childbearing.* Washington, DC.: National Academy Press.

Hecht, R., A. Alban, K. Taylor, S. Post, N. Andersen, and R. Schwarz. (2006). "Putting it Together: AIDS and the Millennium Development Goals." *PLoS Med* 3(11), November 28.

Heckel, N.I. (1986). *Innovations in Population Law and Policy in Sub-Saharan Africa: 1975–1985.* New York, Columbia University Center for Population and Family Health.

Heggenhougen, K.H. and J.P. Lugalla, eds. (2005). *Social Change and Health in Tanzania*. Dar es Salaam: Dar es Salaam University Press.

Helzner, J. and B. Shepard. (1997). "The Feminist Agenda in Population Private Voluntary Organizations." In *Women, International Development, and Politics: The Bureaucratic Mire*. Ed. Staudt, K. Philadelphia: Temple University Press. pp. 167–184.

Heuveline, Patrick. (2003) "HIV and Population Dynamics: A General Model and Maximum-Likelihood Standards for East Africa." *Demography* 40(2):217–245.

Hodgson, D. (1988) "Orthodoxy and Revisionism in American Demography." *Population and Development Review* (14):541–569.

———. (1983). "Demography as Social Science and Policy Science." *Population and Development Review* (9):1–34.

Hodgson, D. and S.C. Watkins. (1997). "Feminists and Neo-Malthusians: Past and Present Alliances." *Population and Development Review* 23(3):469–523.

Howard, M. (1994). "Socio-Economic Causes and Cultural Explanations of Childhood Malnutrition Among the Chagga of Tanzania." *Social Science and Medicine* 38(2):239–251.

Hunt, N.R. (1999). *A Colonial Lexicon of Birth Ritual, Medicalization, and Mobility in the Congo*. Durham, NC: Duke University Press.

———. (1988). "'Le Bebe en Brousse': European Women, African Birth Spacing and Colonial Intervention in Breast Feeding in the Belgian Congo." *International Journal of African Historical Studies* 21:401–432.

Illich, Ivan. (1993). "Needs." In *The Development Dictionary: A Guide to Knowledge as Power*. Ed. Wolfgang Sachs. Johannesburg and London: Witwatersrand University Press and Zed Books. pp. 88–101.

International Planned Parenthood Federation (IPPF). (1988). *Evaluation of JOICFP Integrated Projects in Tanzanian and Zambia*. London: IPPF.

Jackson, S. (1998). *Britain's Population: Demographic Issues in Contemporary Society*. London and New York: Routledge.

Jacobus, M., E.F. Keller, and S. Shuttleworth. eds. (1990). *Body/Politics: Women and the Discourses of Science*. New York and London: Routledge.

Jain, A. (1998). *Do Population Policies Matter?: Fertility and Politics in Egypt, India, Kenya, and Mexico*. New York: The Population Council.

Johnson-Hanks, J. (2002). "On the Modernity of Traditional Contraception: Time and the Social Context of Fertility." *Population and Development Review* 28(2), June:229–249.

Johnson-Odim, C. (1991). "Common Themes, Different Contexts: Third World Women and Feminism." In *Third World Women and the Politics of Feminism*. Ed. Mohanty, C.H. A. Russo, and L. Torres. Bloomington and Indianapolis: Indiana University Press. pp. 314–327.

Kabeer, N. (1994). *Reversed Realities: Gender Hierarchies in Development Thought*. London and New York: Verso.

Kaler, Amy. (2003). *Running After Pills: Politics, Gender, and Contraception in Colonial Zimbabwe*. Portsmouth NH and London: Heinemann.

Kapiga, S.H., and J.L.P. Lugalla. (2002). "Sexual Behaviour Patterns and Condom Use in Tanzania: Results from the 1996 Demographic and Health Survey." *AIDS Care* 14(4):455–469.

Kaplan, G. (1976). "An Afternoon with Anwar el-Sadat." *Institutional Investor*. August.

Keyfitz, N. (1977). *Applied Mathematical Demography*. New York: Wiley-Interscience, John Wiley and Sons.

Keysers, L. (1999). "The Politics of Inclusion and Exculsion: Fortress Europe and the Reproductive Rights Agenda." *Development* 42(1):18–24.

Kihamia, C.M. and J.J. Maro. (1984). "The UMATI Integrated Family Planning, Nutrition and Parasite Control Project (IP) in Masama & TPC Localities in Moshi District of Kilimanjaro Tanzania: Report on Baseline Data and Preliminary (IP) Activities." Dar es Salaam: UMATI.

Kiondo, A.S.Z. (1995). "When the State Withdraws: Local Development, Politics and Liberalisation in Tanzania." In *Liberalised Development in Tanzania*. Ed. Gibbon, P. Uppsala: Nordic Africa Institute. pp. 109–176.

Kirk, D. (1996). "Demographic Transition Theory." *Population Studies* 50:361–387.

Knowles, J.C., K.A. Bollen, and K. Yount. (1994). *The Policy Environment of Family Planning Programs: A Literature Review. The EVALUATION Project Working Paper*. Chapel Hill, NC: Carolina Population Center.

Knudsen, Lara M. (2006). *Reproductive Rights in a Global Context: South Africa, Uganda, Peru, Denmark, United States, Vietnam, Jordan*. Nashville, TN: Vanderbuilt University Press.

Kon, Y. (1995). Regional Workshop on the Integrated Project (PANFRICO V) Congratulatory Address. PANFRICO V, Dar es Salaam, UMATI.

Kuhlmann, E. and B. Babitsch. (2002). "Bodies, Health, Gender—Bridging Feminist Theories and Women's Health." *Women's Studies International Forum* 25(4):433–442.

Lane, S.D. (1994). "From Population Control to Reproductive Health: An Emerging Policy Agenda." *Social Science and Medicine* 39(9):1303–1314.

Larsen, U. (1997). "Fertility in Tanzania: Do Contraception and Sub-Fertility Matter?" *Population Studies* 51:213–220.

Lenga, B. (1987). *Tanzania Faces Up to Its Population Boom*. GE 8883. London: Gemini News Service.

Lewis-Jones, H. (1980). "Statement by Ms. Helen Lewis-Jones UNFPA Coordinator in Dar es Salaam to the National Seminar on Population and Development—Arusha 17–24 February 1980." In *Final Report on the National Seminar on Population and Development in the United Republic of Tanzania*. Ed. Economic Commission for Africa/International Labour Organisation Arusha: UNFPA. pp. 187–191.

Lloyd, C.B., C.E. Kaufman, and Hewett. (1999). *The Spread of Primary Schooling in Sub-Saharan Africa*. New York: The Population Council.

Lock, M. and N. Scheper-Hughes. (1996). "A Critical-Interpretive Approach in Medical Anthropology: Rituals and Routines of Discipline and Dissent." In *Medical Anthropology: Contemporary Theory and Method Revised Edition*. Ed. Sargent, C.F. and T.M. Johnson. Westport, CT and London: Praeger, pp. 21–40.

Lock, M. and P.A. Kaufert. (1998). *Pragmatic Women and Body Politics*. New York and Cambridge: Cambridge University Press.

Luke, N. and S.C. Watkins. (2002). "Reactions of National Elites to International Population Policy." Population and Development Review 28(4):707–733.

Lykke, N. and R. Braidotti. eds. (1996). *Between Monsters, Goddesses and Cyborgs: Feminist Confrontations with Science, Medicine and Cyberspace.* London: Zed Books.

Makinson, C. (1985). "The Health Consequences of Teenage Fertility." Family Planning *Perspectives* (17):132–139.

Malima, K.A. (1980). "Speech by Prof. K.A. Malima, Minister of State for Planning and Economic Affairs at the Opening of the National Seminar on Population and Development in Arusha, 18 February 1980." In *Final Report on the National Seminar on Population and Development in the United Republic of Tanzania*. Ed. Economic Commission for Africa/International Labour Organisation Arusha: UNFPA. pp. 169–173.

Malthus, T.R. (1914). *An Essay on Population.* New York: E.P. Dutton and Co.

Mansuri, D. (1998). "Solicitation for PSC Health Sector Advisor. USAID," www.info.usaid.gov/ftp_data/pub/OP/PSC/ accessed on November 10, 1998.

Mauldin, W.P. and J.A. Ross. (1989). "Historical Perspectives on the Introduction of Contraceptive Technology." In *Demographic and Programmatic Consequences of Contraceptive Innovations.* Ed. Segal, S.J., A.O. Tsui, and S.M. Rogers. New York: Plenum Press. pp. 33–52.

Mburu, F.M. (1995). *Update on The Family Planning Services Support Project: Tanzania Socioeconomic Environment, Status and Prospects for Family Planning Services.* Dar es Salaam: USAID.

McNicoll, G. (1992). "The Agenda of Population Studies: A Commentary and Complaint." *Population and Development Review* 18:399–420.

Mercer, C. (1999). "Power, Participation and Development on Mount Kilimanjaro: The Non-Governmental Sector and the State in Tanzania." PhD Thesis, Department of Geography, Liverpool, University of Liverpool.

Mkini, A.H. (1995). Background Paper on Integrated Project in Morogoro Region. In *PANFRICO V.* Dar es Salaam: UMATI.

———. (1980). "Current Population Policy in the United Republic of Tanzania." In *Final Report on the National Seminar on Population and Development in the United Republic of Tanzania.* Ed. Economic Commission for Africa/International Labour Organisation Arusha: UNFPA. pp. 62–73.

Moffett, G.D. (1994). *Critical Masses: The Global Population Challenge.* New York: Viking.

Mohanty, C.T. (1991). "Introduction: Cartographies of Struggle: Third World Women and the Politics of Feminism." In *Third World Women and The Politics of Feminism.* Ed. Mohanty, C.T., A. Russo, and L. Torres. Bloomington and Indianapolis: Indiana University Press.

Morsy, S.A. (1995). "Deadly Reproduction among Egyptian Women: Maternal Mortality and the Medicalization of Population Control." In *Conceiving the New World Order: The Global Politics of Reproduction.* Ed. Ginsburg, F.D and R. Rapp. Berkeley: University of California Press. pp. 162–176.

Mosha, E.R. (1994). *Report on UMATI/JOICFP Community Based Distribution of Family Planning Services Workshop Mlali Ward, Morogoro From 12 December to 30 December 1994.* Morogoro, Tanzania: IDM-Mzumbe.

Mpangile, G.S. (1994). *Review of the 1989–1993 Plan of Operations of the National Family Planning Program.* Dar es Salaam: World Bank.

Mpango wa Taifa wa Uzazi wa Mpango na Afya ya Uzazi. (1997). Wizara ya Afya [National Family Planning and Reproductive Health Program]. Mpango wa Kusambaza Huduma za Uzazi wa Mpango na Afya ya Uzazi kwa Kuhusisha Jamii Tanzania: Mwongozo wa Mhudumu. Dar es Salaam: MOH and Pathfinder International.

Narayan, U.L. (1997). *Dislocating Cultures: Identities, Traditions and third world Feminism.* London and New York: Routledge.

National Bureau of Statistics, Tanzania and Macro International Inc. (2000). *Tanzania Reproductive and Child Health Survey 1999.* Calverton, MD: Macro International Inc.

National Bureau of Statistics, Tanzania and MEASURE Evaluation. (2000). *Tanzania Reproductive and Child Health Facility Survey, 1999.* Dar es Salaam: MEASURE Evaluation Technical Report Series No. 7.

Ngallaba, S., S.H. Kapiga, I. Ruyobya, and J.T. Boerma. (1991/1992). *Tanzania Demographic* and Health Survey 1991/1992. Columbia, MA: Macro International.

Notestein, F.W. (1982). "Demography in the United States: A Partial Account of the Development of the Field." *Population and Development Review* 8(65):1–87.

Ntukula, M. (1994). "The Initiation Rite." In *Chelewa, Chelwa: The Dilemma of Teenage Girls.* Ed. Tumbo-Masabo, Z and R. Liljestrom. Stockholm: The Scandinavian Institute of African Studies. pp. 96–120.

Nsekela, C.M.K. (1985). Parliamentarians Seminar April 27–30, 1985—Dodoma, Tanzania.

Nyerere, J.K. (1973). *Freedom and Development/Uhuru na Maendeleo.* Dar es Salaam: Oxford University Press.

Okunnu, M.A. (1995). "Statement by Mr. Marc A. Okunnu, Sr, Regional Director, IPPF Africa Region at the Opening Ceremony of the Fifth Pan African Conference (PANFRICO) on the Integrated Nutrition, Parasite Control and Family Planning Project (IP), Dar es Salaam, 5th December, 1995." In *PANFRICO V.* Dar es Salaam (speech transcript).

———. (1992). *Report on the First Meeting of Participating Agencies in the Tanzania National Family Planning Programme.* Morogoro Hotel, Morogoro Tanzania: JSI/SEATS Project for the FPU, MOH.

Oliff, M., P. Mayaud, R. Brugha, and A.M. Semakafu. (2003). "Integrating Reproductive Health Services in a Reforming Health Sector: The Case of Tanzania." *Reproductive Health Matters* 11(21): 37–48.

Omari, C.K. (1989). *Social-Cultural Factors in Modern Family Planning Methods in Tanzania.* Wales, UK: The Edwin Mellen Press.

Oosterhuis, A. (1989). "The Promotion Of Family Planning In Tanzania: Context, Structure And Reception Of Written Promotion Material." doctoraalscriptie (thesis).

Oudshoorn, N. (1996). "The Decline of the One-Size-Fits-All Paradigm, Or, How Reproductive Scientists Try to Cope With Postmodernity." In *Between Monsters, Goddesses and Cyborgs: Feminist Confrontations with Science,*

Medicine and Cyberspace. Ed. Lykke, N. and R. Braidotti. London: Zed Books. pp. 153–173.

Overseas Development Administration. (1991). *National Policy Environment Report: Overseas Development Administration*. London: Overseas Development Administration.

Palmer, I. (1992). *Gender Equity and Economic Efficiency in Adjustment Models*. London, Macmillan.

Parpart, J.L. (1995). "Post-Modernism, Gender and Development." In *Power of Development*. Ed. J. Crush. London and New York: Routledge. pp. 253–265.

Peterson, V.S. (2002). "Rewriting (Global) Political Economy as Reproductive, Productive, and Virtual (Foucauldian) Economies." *International Feminist Journal of Politics* 4(1):116–121.

Ponte, Stefano. (2002). *Farmers and Markets in Tanzania*. Oxford, Dar es Salaam, and Portsmouth, NH: James Currey, Mkuki na Nyota, Heinemann.

Population Planning Unit, Planning Commission, Bureau of Statistics, and Ministry of Health National Family Planning Programme. (1995). *Population and Development in Tanzania: Presentation and Report*. Dar es Salaam: RAPID IV project.

Potts, M. (1995). "Cairo's Skewed Consensus." *Population Today* 4–5, November. http://www.un.org/popin/popis/journals/poptoday/today1195.html accessed on September 12, 2007.

Presser, H.B. (2000). "Demography, Feminism, and the Science-Policy Nexus." *Women's Empowerment and Demographic Processes: Moving Beyond Cairo*. Ed. Presser and Sen. Oxford and New York, Oxford University Press. pp. 377–412.

———. (1997). "Demography, Feminism, and the Science-Policy Nexus." *Population and Development Review* 23(2), June:295–332.

Presser, H.B. and G. Sen. (2000). *Women's Empowerment and Demographic Processes: Moving Beyond Cairo*. Oxford and New York: Oxford University Press.

Przeworski, A. and H. Teune. (1970). *The Logic of Comparative Social Inquiry*. New York: Wiley-Interscience.

Rabinow, P. (1984). "Introduction." In *The Foucault Reader*. Ed. Rabinow, P. New York: Pantheon Books. pp. 3–31.

Raikes, A. (1992). "Gender and the Production of Health Care Services: Issues for Women's Roles in Health Development." *IDS Bulletin* 23(1):19–28.

Rajani, R. (2002). *Situation Analysis of Children in Tanzania*. New York: UNICEF.

Ramsden, E. (2002). "Carving up Population Science: Eugenics, Demography and the Controversy over the 'Biological Law' of Population Growth." *Social Studies of Science* 32(5/6):857–899.

Rapp, R. (1990). "Constructing Amniocentesis: Maternal and Medical Discourses." In Uncertain *Terms: Negotiating Gender in American Culture*. Ed. Ginsburg and Tsing. Boston: Beacon Press. pp. 28–42.

Reid, S.T. and D.L. Lyon. (1972). *Population Crisis: An Interdisciplinary Perspective*. Glenview, IL: Scott Foresman.

Renne, E.P. and E. Van de Walle. (2001). "Introduction." In *Regulating Menstruation: Beliefs, Practices, Interpretations*. Ed. Renne, E.P and Vande Walle, E. Chicago and London: University of Chicago Press. pp. xiii–xxxix.

Richey, L.A. (2004). "From the Policies to the Clinics: The Reproductive Health Paradox in Post-Adjustment Health Care." *World Development* 32(6):923–940.

———. (2003). "Women's Reproductive Health and Population Policy: A Case Study from Tanzania." *Review of African Political Economy* (96):273–292.

———. (1999). "Family Planning and the Politics of Population in Tanzania: International to Local Discourse." *The Journal of Modern African Studies* 37(3), September:457–487.

Riedmann, Agnes. (1993). Science *that Colonizes: A Critique of Fertility Studies in Africa*. Philadelphia: Temple University Press.

Riley, N.E. and J. McCarthy. (2003). *Demography in the Age of the Postmodern*. Cambridge: Cambridge University Press.

Robins, S. (2003). "Whose Modernity? Indigenous Modernities and Land Claims after Apartheid." *Development and Change* 34(2), April:265–286.

Ross, E.B. (1998). *The Malthus Factor: Poverty, Politics and Population in Capitalist Development*. London and New York, Zed Books.

Rowlands, J. (1998). "A Word of the Times, but what does it mean?: Empowerment in the Discourse and Practice of Development." In *Women and Empowerment: Illustrations from the Third World*. Ed. Afshar, H. New York: St. Martin's Press. pp. 11–34.

Russell, A., E.J. Sobo, and M.S. Thompson. (2000). *Contraception Across Cultures,Technologies, Choices, Constraints*. Oxford and New York: Berg.

Russell, A. and M.S. Thompson. (2000). "Introduction: Contraception across Cultures." In *Contraception Across Cultures. Technologies, Choices, Constraints*. Ed. Russell, A., E.J. Sobo, and M.S. Thompson. Oxford and New York: Berg.

Rutenberg, N. and S.C. Watkins. (1997). "The Buzz Outside the Clinics: Conversations and Contraception in Nyanza Province, Kenya." *Studies in Family Planning* 28(4):290–307.

Sai, F.T. (1988). "Key Issues and Problems in African Population Policy in the 1990's." *African Population Conference* IUSSP. 3, November 7–12:21–36.

Scheper-Hughes, N. (1997). "Demography Without Numbers." *Anthropological Demography: Toward a New Synthesis*. Eds. Kertzer, D.I. and T. Fricke. Chicago: University of Chicago Press.

Scott, J.C. (1998). *Seeing the State: How Certain Schemes to Improve the Human Condition have Failed*. New Haven, CT: Yale University Press.

———. (1985). *Weapons of the Weak: Everyday Forms of Peasant Resistance*. New Haven: Yale University Press.

Sembajwe, I.S.L. (1984). *Population and Development: With Special Reference to Tanzania*. Arusha: Institute of Resource Assessment, UDSM.

Semina Juu ya Idadi ya Watu na Maendeleo. (1985). "Seminar on Population and Development: Maazimio (Declarations)." *Semina Juu ya Idadi ya Watu na Maendeleo*. Taasisi ys Saruji; Dar es Salaam.

Sen, A. (1995). "Food and Freedom." In *Development Studies: A Reader*. Ed. Corbridge, S. New York: John Wiley and Sons. pp. 90–108.

Sen, G. (1994). "Development, Population, and the Environment: A Search for Balance." In *Population Policies Reconsidered: Health, Empowerment and Rights*. Ed. Sen, G., A. Germain, and L.C. Chen. Boston: Harvard University Press. pp. 63–74.

Sen, G. and S. Batliwala. (2000). "Empowering Women for Reproductive Rights." *Women's Empowerment and Demographic Processes: Moving Beyond Cairo*. Ed. Presser H.B. and G. Sen. London and New York, Oxford University Press. pp. 15–36.

Setel, P.W. (1999). *A Plague of Paradoxes: AIDS, Culture, and Demography in Northern Tanzania*. Chicago and London: University of Chicago Press.

———. (1995). "The Social Context of AIDS Education among Young Men in Northern Kilimanjaro." In *Young People at Risk: Fighting AIDS in Northern Tanzania*.Ed. Klepp, K.I., P.M. Biswalo, and A. Talle. Oslo: Scandinavian University Press. pp. 49–68.

Sharpless, J. (1997). "Population Science, Private Foundations, and Development Aid: The Transformation of Demographic Knowledge in the United States, 1945–1965." In *International Development and the Social Sciences*. Ed. Cooper, F. and R. Packard. Berkeley: University of California Press. pp. 176–200.

Silliman, J. and Y. King, eds. (1999). *Dangerous Intersections: Feminist Perspectives on Population, Environment, and Development*. Cambridge, MA: South End Press.

Sinding, S. and J. Caldwell. (1997). "Where is the International Population Movement Going? Cairo's Legacy." Supplement four to *Health Transition Review* 7.

Spallone, P. and D.L. Steinberg. (1987). *Made to Order: The Myth of Reproductive and Genetic Progress*. Oxford and New York: Pergamon Press.

Speizer, I.S., D.R. Hotchkiss, R.J. Magnani, B. Hubbard, and K. Nelson. (2000). "Do Service Providers in Tanzania Unnecessarily Restrict Clients' Access to Contraceptive Methods?" *International Family Planning Perspectives* 26(1):13–20.

Stamp, P. (1990). *Technology, Gender and Power in Africa*. Ottawa: International Development Research Centre.

Standing, H. (2002). *Towards Equitable Financing Strategies for Reproductive Health* IDS Working Paper No. 153, Brighton: IDS Sussex.

Stanecki, K.A. (2002). *The AIDS Pandemic in the 21st Century*. Barcelona, USAID and US Census Bureau.

Staudt, K. (1991). *Managing Development: State, Society, and International Contexts*. Newbury Park, CA: Sage Publications, Inc.

Szreter, S.R.S. (1993). "The Idea of Demographic Transition: a Critical Intellectual History." *Population and Development Review* (19):659–701.

Tanzania Bureau of Statistics, Planning Commission. (2000). *Tanzania Reproductive and Child Health Survey (1999)*. Calverton, MD: Macro Int.

Tanzania Food and Nutrition Centre. (1995). *Nutrition Situation Analysis on Integrated Family Planning, Nutrition and Parasite Control Project in Morogoro and Kilimanjaro Regions June–August 1993*. Dar es Salaam: Tanzania Food and Nutrition Centre and UMATI.

Tanzanian Ministry of Health Reproductive Health Unit National Family Planning Programme. (1999). *Annual Report Jan–Dec 1998*. Dar es Salaam, MOH.

Tesfaye, M. (2003). *Cultural Spaces, Habitats of Power: Smallholders, Local Community and the "Modernizing" State in Warahimanu, Wollo, Ethiopia*. PhD Dissertation, Department of Anthropology, Urbana-Champaign, University of Illinois.

Thomas, I. (1979). "Population Policy in Tanzania." Norwich, UK: University of East Anglia, School of Development Studies.

Thomas, J.W. and M.S. Grindle. (1994). "Political Leadership and Policy Characteristics in Population Policy Reform." *Population and Development Review* 20(Suppl.on The New Politics of Population: Conflict and Consensus in Family Planning):51–70.

Tilly, C. (1999). "Survey Article: Power -Top Down and Bottom Up." *The Journal of Political Philosophy* 7(3):330–352.

Tumbo-Masabo, Z. (1994). "Conclusions." In *Chelewa, Chelewa: The Dilemma of Teenage Girls*. Ed. Tumbo-Masabo, Z. and R. Liljestrom. Stockholm: The Scandinavian Institute of African Studies.

Turshen, M. (1987). "Population Growth and the Deterioration of Health: Mainland Tanzania 1920–1960." In *African Population and Capitalism: Historical Perspectives*. Ed. Cordell, D.D. and G.W. Gregory. Boulder, CO: Westview Press.

Uganda Ministry of Health. (1999). *Sexual and Reproductive Health, Minimum Package for Uganda. Kampala*. Uganda Ministry of Health.

UMATI. (1996). Three Year Plan 1996–1998. Dar es Salaam: UMATI.

———. (1995a). The Integrated Family Planning, Nutrition and Parasite Control Project: Tanzania Country Paper. In *PANFRICO V*. Dar es Salaam.

———. (1995b). The Annual Workshop on the Integrated Parasite Control, Nutrition and Family Planning Project (IP) in Tanzania. Morogoro, Tanzania: UMATI.

———. (1995c). Integrated Project (IP) Data Review. In *PANFRICO V*. Dar es Salaam: UMATI.

———. (1995d). From file of IPPF London: as submitted by UMATI three-year plan (1996–1998); Dar es Salaam April 1995 .

———. (1993). Three Year Plan 1993–1995. Dar es Salaam: UMATI.

———. (1992). Towards Meeting Future Challenges in Family Planning. Morogoro, Tanzania: UMATI.

———. (1984). Information Sheet for Participants to the Members of Parliament Seminar to be Held in Arusha during May 10–14, 1984.

UNAIDS. Joint United Nations Programme on HIV/AIDS. (2000). "The United Nations on the Demographic Impact of the AIDS Epidemic." *Population and Development Review* 26(3):629–633.

United Nations Economic Commission for Africa. (1993). "An Assessment of the Formulation and Implementation of National Population Programmes in ECA Member States during the 1990s." Addis Ababa, Ethiopia: UNECA.

UNAIDS. (1992). "Third African Population Conference Country Reports." Dakar, Senegal: UNECA.

UNAIDS. (1990). "Population Issues for ECA Member States During the 1990s." Tripoli, Libya: UNECA.

———. (1989). *African Population Studies Series Number 10: Status and Prospects of Population Policies in ECA Member States*. New York: United Nations.

UNAIDS. (1984). "Report of the Second African Population Conference." In *Second African Population Conference*. Arusha, Tanzania: United Nations Economic Commission for Africa.

United Nations Population Fund. (1979). United Republic of Tanzania: Report of Mission on Needs Assessment for Population Assistance. New York: UNFPA.

———. (1994a). Project Agreement between the Government of The United Republic of Tanzania and the United Nations Population Fund Project Number URT/95/P10 Population Planning Unit. Dar es Salaam: UNFPA.

———. (1994b). UNFPA United Nations Population Fund in Tanzania: Commemorating 25 years of Dedication to Population Assistance. Dar es Salaam: UNFPA.

———. (1994c). UNFPA Third Country Programme 1992–1996 Mid-Term Review Report. Dar es Salaam: UNFPA.

———. (1994d). *Quality of Family Planning Services*. New York: UNFPA.

———. (1994e). UNF Third Country Program 1992–1996 Mid-Term Review Report. Dar es Salaam: UNFPA

United Republic of Tanzania. (1994). Country Report on Population and Development to the International Conference on Population and Development to be held in Cairo, Egypt September 5–13, 1994. Dar es Salaam.

———. (1992). *The National Population Policy*. Dar es Salaam: The Planning Commission of the President's Office.

———. (1991). Developments in Policy and Institutional Reforms Since December 1989: Report prepared by the Government of Tanzania for the Meeting of the Consultative Group for Tanzania Paris, June 1991. Dar es Salaam.

———. (1989). Economic Recovery Programme II 1989/90–1991/92: Report prepared by the Government of Tanzania for the Meeting of the Consultative Group for Tanzania Paris, December 1989. Dar es Salaam.

———. (1988). Programme for Economic Recovery: Report prepared by the Government of Tanzania for the Meeting of the Consultative Group for Tanzania, Paris, July 1988. Dar es Salaam.

———. (1985). Tanzania Government Programme for Economic Recovery. Dar es Salaam.

United Republic of Tanzania, Ministry of Community Development Women Affairs and Children. (1992). Brief of Population/Family Life Education Programme (POPFLEP). Morogoro, Tanzania: MCDWC.

United Republic of Tanzania, Ministry of Health. (1994a). National Family Planning Programme Strategic Plan July 1994–June 1999. Dar es Salaam: MOH.

———. (1994b). National Family Planning Programme Annual Report January–December 1994. Dar es Salaam, Tanzania: MOH.

———. (1993a). National Family Planning Programme Tripartite Review Meeting. Dar es Salaam: Ministry of Health.

———. (1993b). Family Planning Programme Annual Report 1993. Dar es Salaam, Tanzania: FPU/MOH.

———. (1992). National Family Planning Programme Annual Report 1992. Dar es Salaam, Tanzania: MOH.

United Republic of Tanzania, Ministry of Health and Social Welfare. (1989). The National Family Planning Programme Plan of Operations 1989–1993. Dar es Salaam: MOH.

Upunda. (1995). "Keynote Speech: IP Experience, Present Status and Situational Analysis in Tanzania." In *PANFRICO V.* Dar es Salaam.

Urrio, T. (1995). "IP Development in Tanzania." In The Regional Workshop on the Integrated Project (*PANFRICO V*). Dar es Salaam: UMATI.

———. (1984). "The Linkages between Family Planning, Family Health and National Development." Arusha, Tanzania.

USAID. (1994). *Midterm Review of the Tanzania Family Planning Services Support (FPSS) Project. Arlington.* VA: Population and Technical Assistance Project.

———. (1990). Project Paper: Family Planning Services Support. Dar es Salaam: USAID.

Van de Kaa, D.J. (1996). "Anchored Narratives: the Story and Findings of Half a Century of Research into the Determinants of Fertility." *Population Studies* 50(3):389–432.

———. (1987). "The Cairo Conference: A Demographer's View."In *Population and Family in the Low Countries.* Ed. van den Brekel, H., and F. Deven. Dordrecht, Boston, and London: Kluwer Academic Pub. pp. 21–39.

Van Eeuwijk, B.O. and S. Mlangwa. (1997). "Competing Ideologies: Adolescence, Knowledge and Silences in Dar es Salaam." In *Power, Reproduction and Gender: The Intergenerational Transfer of Knowledge.* Ed. W. Harcourt. London: Zed Books. pp. 35–57.

Vaughan, M. (1991). *Curing their Ills: Colonial Power and African Illness.* Cambridge: Polity Press.

Vavrus, Frances. (2003). *Desire and Decline: Schooling amid Crisis in Tanzania.* New York: Peter Lang Publishers.

Vavrus, F. and L. Richey. (2003). "Women and development: rethinking policy and reconceptualizing practice." In Frances Vavrus, Lisa Ann Richey (eds), *Rethinking policy and conceptualizing practice*, Eds. Vavrus, F. and L. Richey. New York: The Feminist Press. (Women's studies quarterly) 31. pp. 6–18.

Verba, S. (1967). "Some Dilemmas of Comparative Research." *World Politics* (20):111–128.

Viederman, S. (1980). "Statement by Mr. S. Viederman UNFPA Headquarters." In *Final Report on the National Seminar on Population and Development in the United Republic of Tanzania.* Ed. Economic Commission for Africa/ International Labour Organisation: UNFPA. Arusha. pp. 192–201.

Ward, M.C. (1995). "Early Childbearing: What Is the Problem and Who Owns It?" In *Conceiving the New World Order: The Global Politics of Reproduction.* Eds. Ginsburg and Rapp. Berkeley: University of California Press. pp. 140–158.

Warwick, D.P. (1982). *Bitter Pills: Population Policies and Their Implementation in Eight Developing Countries.* Cambridge: Cambridge University Press.

Watkins, S.C. (2000). "Local and Foreign Models of Reproduction in Nyanza Province, Kenya, 1930–1998." *Population and Development Review* 26(4):725–759.

———. (1998). "Local Transformations in Reproductive Ideologies in a Global Context 1930–1997." Paper prepared for a Rockefeller Foundation Meeting, Bellagio May 18–22, 1998.

Watkins, S.C. (1993). "If All We Knew About Women Was What We Read in *Demography*, What Would We Know?" *Demography* 30(4):551–577.

Watkins, S.C., N. Rutenberg, and D. Wilkinson. (1997). "Orderly Theories, Disorderly Women." In *The Continuing Demographic Transition.* Ed. Jones, G.W., R.M.J. Douglas, J.C. Caldwell, and R.M. D'Souza. Oxford, Clarendon Press. pp. 213–245.

Weber, M. (1978). *Economy and Society.* Berkeley: University of California Press (first published 1922).

Weinstein, K.I., S. Ngallaba, A.R. Cross, and F.M. Mburu. (1995). *Tanzania: Knowledge, Attitudes and Practices Survey 1994.* Calverton, Maryland: Macro International.

Whelpton, P.K. and C.V. Kiser, eds. (1946–1958). *Social and Psychological Factors Affecting Fertility*, 5 vols. New York: Milbank Memorial Fund.

Whiteford, L.M. and L. Mandeson. (2000). *Global Health Policy, Local Realities: The Fallacy of the Level Playing Field.* Boulder and London: Lynne Rienner.

Wieringa, S. (1994). "Women's Interests and Empowerment: Gender Planning Reconsidered." *Development and Change* 25:849–878.

Williams, G. (1995). "Modernizing Malthus: The World Bank, Population Control and the African Environment." In *Power of Development.* Ed. Crush, J. New York and London: Routledge. pp. 158–175.

Wilson, C. (2001). "On the Scale of Global Demographic Convergence 1950–2000." *Population and Development Review* 27(1):155–171.

Wolf, E.R. (1999). *Envisioning Power, Ideologies of Dominance and Crisis.* Berkeley: University of California Press.

———. (1969). *Peasant Wars of the Twentieth Century.* New York: Harper and Row.

World Bank. (1996). From Plan to Market: World Development Report 1996. Oxford: Oxford University Press.

———. (1994). Population and Development: Implications for the World Bank. Washington, DC: The World Bank.

———. (1989). Report to the Consultative Group for Tanzania on The Government's Economic and Social Policy Reform Program: The World Bank Southern Africa Department.

———. (1986). Consultative Group for Tanzania Paris June 10–11, 1986: Statement on World Bank Assistance. Paris: World Bank.

———. (1988). Meeting of Consultative Group for Tanzania: Current Economic Developments and Future Prospects.

Worrall, J. (1983). "East Africans Urged to Accept Family Planning." *Africa*:28–29.

Yanoshik, K. and J. Norsigian. (1989). "Contraception, Control and Choice: International Perspectives." In: *Healing technology: feminist perspectives*, edited by K. S. Ratcliff, M. M. Ferree, G. O. Mellow, B. D. Wright, G. D. Price, K. Yanoshik, M. S. Freston. Ann Arbor, Michigan: University of Michigan. pp. 61–92.

Yuval-Davies. 1994. "Women, Ethnicity and Empowerment." *Feminism and Psychology* 4(1):179–197.

Zeleza, P.T. (1997). *Manufacturing African Studies and Crises*. Dakar, Senegal: CODESRIA.

Zelizer, V. and A. Rotman. (1985). *Pricing the Priceless Child : The Changing Social Value of Children*. New York: Basic Books.

———. (1979). *Morals and Markets. The Development of Life Insurance in the United States*. New York: Columbia University Press.

Index